THE HUMAN FUEL HANDBOOK

Nutrition for Peak Athletic Performance

From Health For Life

Also by **Health For Life***:*

- **Legendary Abs**

- **Beyond Legendary Abs**
  A synergistic performance guide to Legendary Abs and SynerAbs

- **Power ForeArms!**

- **Maximum Calves**

- **SynerAbs:** 6 Minutes to a Flatter Stomach

- **SynerShape:** A Scientific Weight Loss Guide

- **SynerStretch:** For Whole Body Flexibility

- **The Psychology of Weight Loss:**
  A Guided Introspection

- **Secrets of Advanced Bodybuilders**
  A manual of synergistic weight training for the whole body

- **Secrets of Advanced Bodybuilders, Supplement #1**

Library of Congress Catalog #88-138994   ISBN 0-944831-17-6

Health For Life
8033 Sunset Blvd.
Suite 483
Los Angeles, CA 90046
(213) 450-0070

10 9 8 7 6 5 4 3

CONTENTS

PART THREE: BAD NUTRITION

PART FOUR: NUTRITION AND ATHLETIC PERFORMANCE

PART FIVE: SIX NUTRITIONAL PROGRAMS FOR PEAK ATHLETIC PERFORMANCE

INTRODUCTION

INTRODUCTION

Finally, the ultimate nutrition program!

The Human Fuel Handbook is a comprehensive approach to sports nutrition. It brings together the most sophisticated nutritional information available and synthesizes it into proven, effective programs for all athletes—from bodybuilders to triathletes (and everyone in between).

The book begins by explaining the physiological basis for athletic nutrition. Nutrient by nutrient, it examines *how* protein, carbohydrate, fat, minerals, and vitamins function in your body, and *why* much of what you've heard about these substances is wrong.

Next, **The Handbook** explores the many ways good nutrition goes bad. It exposes deceptive business practices designed to misinform you for profit. It explodes the fallacies behind a number of popular nutritional fads. And it takes a hard look at drugs that may improve your performance but destroy your health.

Following this excursion into nutrition's darker side, **The Handbook** examines optimum nutrition for athletic performance, including a detailed look at energy production, sports drinks, and ergogenic aids (arginine/ornithine, octacosanol, *Eleutherococcus*, and others—which ones work, which don't).

Finally, **The Handbook** lays out detailed nutritional programs. No matter if you are a bodybuilder, martial artist, marathoner, or weekend racquetball player, you will find in Part Five the key to optimum performance.

HOW TO USE THIS BOOK

The Handbook is designed to be read from cover to cover. The information unfolds in a logical progression, each new area building on what preceded it. If you have the inclination, straight through is the way to go.

On the other hand, you can open **The Handbook** anywhere and start reading—it will refer you to other chapters as necessary.

A third option is to go right to the end and put one of the five programs directly into action.

No matter how you use it, we guarantee **The Human Fuel Handbook** will take your athletic performance to levels you never thought possible!

❖   ❖   ❖

PART ONE

A STARTING PLACE

You've seen the ads:

"Since XYZ directly increases [fill in the blank: muscle growth, definition, endurance, recovery, weight gain, weight loss], taking XYZ supplements will improve your performance!"

This kind of nutritional advice **sounds great.** *The rationale seems to "prove" that XYZ supplements have an impact on your performance. But do they?*

Sometimes yes, sometimes no.

How can you tell? By what yardstick can you evaluate these claims, and separate the fact from the fraud? You need to begin with an understanding of three basic physiological realities: **the digestive system, homeostasis,** *and* **limiting factors.**

A QUICK TRIP THROUGH THE DIGESTIVE SYSTEM

"Unquiet meals make ill digestions."
—William Shakespeare, *The Comedy of Errors*

We can't get very far talking about sports nutrition without at least a brief look at how your body handles what you eat. So let's follow a bite of food from fork to flush.

IN YOUR MOUTH

A forkful of food—say, lasagna—enters your mouth. It is a mouthwatering bite, so your mouth is already watering; that is, saliva flows into your mouth from your **salivary glands**.

The salivary glands are located under your tongue, under your jaw, and in front of your ears. They produce a watery fluid (saliva) that moistens your food and makes it easier to swallow.

But saliva contains more than just water. It also contains an enzyme, **amylase** (also called **ptyalin**) that starts to break down the starches in the lasagna. Meanwhile, the teeth mash the food and the tongue moves it around in your mouth, thoroughly mixing the saliva through the food.

This mashed, moistened, masticated mouthful is then swallowed and slides down the **esophagus**, the tube that connects the mouth with the stomach.

IN YOUR STOMACH

After spending a few seconds in the esophagus, the food enters the **stomach**. The stomach contains a fluid, **gastric juice**, that assists with the next step in digestion. Gastric juice is highly acidic. How acidic? Acidity is measured on what's called the **pH scale**, with lower pH's being more acidic than higher pH's. A pH of 7.0 is "neutral." Gastric juice has a pH of about 1.6, which makes it *almost a million times more acidic than blood (pH 7.4).*

This acid, **hydrochloric acid**, is secreted by cells in the lining of the stomach. Hydrochloric acid does two things: it kills bacteria that enter the stomach with your food, and it provides an acidic environment for the protein-digesting enzyme **pepsin** to work in (pepsin works only in an acidic environment).* The stomach has loops of muscle tissue in its walls which provide a churning action, thoroughly mixing acid and pepsin throughout the stomach contents.

In the stomach, proteins and carbohydrates are partially digested; fats are digested hardly at all.

The stomach has several other functions besides mixing food with acid and pepsin. The stomach facilitates absorption of **iron** and **calcium**, because iron and calcium are better absorbed after having been through an acidic environment. The stomach also produces a protein necessary for the absorption of **vitamin B12** in the small intestine.

The stomach also controls the rate at which the food moves on to the small intestine. It does this by means of a valve at the far end of the stomach, the **pyloric valve**.

So, what has happened to our bite of lasagna in the stomach? The amylase from the salivary glands continued to digest some of the pasta starches until the mouthful hit the stomach acid. The acid made the amylase stop working, but provided a favorable environment for the enzyme *pepsin* to work in. The pepsin "snipped" the long protein chains into smaller chains, and the loops of muscle in the walls of the stomach made sure everything was thoroughly mixed. The fat from the meat and cheese remained pretty much untouched.

What not long ago was a bite of lasagna is now ready to proceed to the small intestine. Food that has been digested to

---

*Most people think it's the stomach acid itself that does the digesting, but this is not true; hydrochloric acid does very little digesting.

this point is now called **chyme** (pronounced *kime*; rhymes with *time*).

The pyloric valve makes sure only a little chyme gets through to the small intestine at a time. Because of this, the pyloric valve is really what's responsible for making you feel full. Since you can put food into your stomach much faster than your pyloric valve will let it out, food tends to *back up* in your stomach and make your stomach more and more full. When your stomach reaches a certain degree of fullness, it sends a message to your brain that the stomach is full and you ought not be hungry anymore.

Chyme containing a lot of fat greatly slows down the rate at which the pyloric valve will let the stomach empty. This is why a fatty meal (or a fatty dessert) fills you up so quickly. The fat slows down the rate of stomach emptying so much that your stomach fills up fast. It's also the reason for the well-known *two-hours-later-and-you're-hungry-again* syndrome of Chinese food. Chinese food (with the exception of the deep-fried stuff) tends to have a lot of vegetables and not much fat. So there's little fat to slow the emptying of the stomach, and your stomach doesn't stay full for long.

Other foods slow down the rate at which the pyloric valve will let the stomach empty, too. These include simple sugars and free form amino acids.

Notice we haven't said anything about absorption. That's because very little absorption takes place in the stomach. Only a few substances, such as alcohol and aspirin, get absorbed in the stomach. Food doesn't get absorbed, for two reasons:

■ the protein, carbohydrates, and fat have not been digested well enough in the stomach to be absorbable

■ the stomach lining is not the right kind of tissue for food absorption anyway.

IN YOUR SMALL INTESTINE

On to the small intestine! The pyloric valve lets a little bit of chyme into the **duodenum**, the first part of the small intestine. This chyme is acidic, because it has lots of acid from the stomach mixed in.

The first order of business of the duodenum is to neutralize the acid. Conveniently, a few inches into the duodenum there is a duct that empties **pancreatic juice** from the **pancreas** and **bile** from the **gall bladder**.

Pancreatic juice contains a lot of **bicarbonate**, an alkaline substance that quickly neutralizes the acid chyme. Pancreatic juice also contains digestive enzymes that continue to break down protein and carbohydrates.

Bile goes to work on the fat. Bile is made in the **liver**, and stored and concentrated in the **gall bladder**. When fat enters the duodenum, the gall bladder squeezes, squirting some bile into the duodenum where the fat is. Bile breaks up the fat into droplets tiny enough to be absorbed through the wall of the intestine.

Meanwhile, enzymes in the pancreatic juice and in the walls of the small intestine have "snipped" the long protein chains into tiny absorbable lengths, and broken the big starch molecules into single sugar units. (More on proteins, carbohydrates, and fats in their respective chapters.) These get absorbed through the walls of the duodenum and the next part of the small intestine, the **jejunum**.

The small intestine consist of three parts: the **duodenum**, the **jejunum**, and the **ileum**. All told, the small intestine is about ten feet long. Nonetheless, virtually all the protein, carbohydrate, fat, minerals, and vitamins are absorbed in the first three feet. The next seven feet or so of the small intestine are there as "reserve," but rarely are needed for that. Mostly that seven feet or so concerns itself with absorption of water, **electrolytes** (sodium, potassium, chloride, and bicarbonate), bile (which gets rechanneled back to the gall bladder and recycled over and over again), and vitamin B12.

IN THE COLON

By the time we get to the **colon** (also called **large intestine**), what's left?

Not much. Virtually all the protein, fat, carbohydrates, minerals, vitamins, and bile have been absorbed already.

Left over we have water, some electrolytes, fiber, and cells from the lining of the digestive system that have been sloughed off along the way. This material becomes fodder for the billions and billions of bacteria that live in your colon.

It's taken about two hours for (what's left of) our bite of lasagna to reach the end of the small intestine/beginning of the colon. It will take another two to three days to see daylight.

The main purpose of the colon is absorption of water and storage of waste matter until a convenient time for disposal. Certain types of carbohydrate (most notably **stachyose** and **raffinose**, found in beans) are not digested in the small intestine but rather fermented by the bacteria in the colon.

This produces some familiar intestinal gases that find their way out into the environment, not always at convenient times.

CONCLUSION

On an average day, you take in about three quarts (six pounds) of water, over a quarter-pound of fat (equal to *more than a whole stick of butter*), about a fifth of a pound of protein, and about three-quarters of a pound of carbohydrates. Total: over seven pounds of food and water.

What finally comes out in the end is less than a half-pound of waste, over a quarter-pound of which is bacteria. Almost no fat, protein, or carbohydrate is left, with the exception of the carbohydrate in indigestible fiber.

"All's well that ends well."
—William Shakespeare, *All's Well That Ends Well*

❖   ❖   ❖

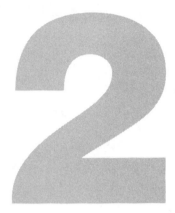

HOMEOSTASIS

An astonishing number of chemical reactions take place in your body simultaneously. These reactions can only transpire if your body provides the appropriate environment for them to do so.

To provide this environment, your body must fine-tune a whole host of factors on a moment-to-moment basis. Each of these factors must remain within narrow boundaries for this appropriate environment to exist. This ongoing *fine-tuning* that provides the appropriate environment for all these chemical reactions is called **homeostasis**.

Some factors that are a part of the homeostatic process are well known to you—for example, **body temperature**.

The myriad chemical reactions that take place in your body work most precisely at a temperature of 98.6 degrees. At temperatures even a little higher or a little lower the reactions become less efficient and less well-controlled.

Your body has a number of compensatory mechanisms for keeping your body temperature remarkably close to 98.6 all the time. These mechanisms include shivering, sweating, opening or closing blood vessels just under the skin to lose or conserve heat, and behavioral changes such as making you want to put on or take off your sweater. You're not aware of them most of the time, but tiny temperature adjustments are going on constantly. Because of all of these temperature control mechanisms, your body maintains a temperature very close to ideal.

Temperature is only one of many factors under homeostatic control. Others include:

- pH—the degree of acidity/alkalinity in your blood and tissues
- blood oxygen level
- blood carbon dioxide level
- blood mineral concentrations—calcium, iron, zinc, and others—your body takes what it needs and stores or discards the rest
- blood vitamin concentrations—vitamin A, B complex, C, D, E, K—your body uses what it needs and stores or discards the rest
- blood glucose (sugar) level
- hormone concentrations—insulin, growth hormone, androgens (male hormones), estrogens (female hormones), thyroid hormones
- protein—your body uses what it needs and discards the rest
- salt concentration
- water content
- blood hemoglobin concentration

Your body does an extraordinarily fine job of balancing all these blood levels and concentrations and many more—a much better job than you ever could if you had to consciously control all these things yourself.

Some of these processes are under tighter homeostatic control than others. The amount of oxygen in your blood, for instance, is tightly controlled: it can vary from ideal levels for only a matter of seconds before compensatory mechanisms restore ideal levels. On the other hand, blood glucose can remain elevated for hours after eating, before compensatory mechanisms restore ideal levels. In general, nutritional levels tend to be among the least tightly-controlled homeostatic processes.

Why is this important?

Peak performance is facilitated by allowing homeostatic mechanisms to work their best. By supplying your body with nutrients in amounts close to what your body needs, homeostatic mechanisms are optimized. You don't need to supply your body with nutrients in *exactly* the amounts required, but you should be close. Amounts of nutrients greatly short of what your body requires cannot be fully compensated for by homeostatic mechanisms. This results in less-than-optimal homeostasis, which in turn can cause less-than-optimal athletic performance.

On the other hand, amounts of nutrients greatly *in excess* of what your body requires *can* generally be fully compensated for by homeostatic mechanisms.

Many athletes take in large quantities of protein and certain vitamins and minerals, feeling that if a little is good, a lot must be better. By and large, this isn't true. **The body recognizes the excess as excess, and, in attempts to return to the homeostatically desirable levels, simply stores or (much more commonly) discards the excess. The Handbook** will point out a number of instances where attempts to improve athletic performance through supplementation are doomed to failure because of the body's unfailing maintenance of homeostasis.

■ **To maintain the appropriate environment for the many chemical reactions occurring in your body, your body fine- tunes a myriad of factors, including blood sugar level, blood vitamin levels, blood mineral levels, pH, blood oxygen level, blood carbon dioxide level, and many others.**

This ongoing fine-tuning is called *homeostasis*.

■ **Homeostatic mechanisms can compensate for eating *too much* of most nutrients (except where those nutrients are toxic in large quantities).**

■ **Homeostatic mechanisms cannot compensate for eating *too little* of most nutrients, and this can result in less-than-optimum athletic performance.**

■ Guideline for optimum athletic performance:

❑ It is important to eat *enough* of every
nutrient to reach the homeostatically
optimum levels, but any beyond that
amount the body treats as excess and
stores or discards.

❖   ❖   ❖

LIMITING FACTORS

As mentioned in the previous chapter, there are an incredible number of chemical reactions that take place simultaneously in your body. No reaction operates alone; rather, each is part of an intricate chain of chemical reactions.

For example, an amino acid in a molecule of protein in a glass of milk may have to go through several hundred different reactions before coming to rest in, say, a molecule of muscle contractile protein. These reactions include several stages of digestion, several stages of absorption including binding to different carrier proteins, reactions of transport, cell entry and exit, binding to protein construction molecules, and many, many more.

Each of these individual reactions is under some kind of homeostatic control. Furthermore, the whole long sequence of successive reactions is under a kind of control. This control is provided by the **limiting factor**.

Limiting factor refers to the single reaction in the entire reaction sequence that is the slowest, or the one reaction which must take place before any of the others do, or the one nutrient necessary for the whole series to take place. In the same way that a chain is no stronger than its weakest link, a chain of reactions cannot proceed without "satisfying" the limiting factor.

This is important because, just like homeostasis, *limiting factors greatly lessen the amount you can externally change a set of physiologic processes*. **In other words, the presence of a limiting factor in every reaction sequence limits how much you can change your body nutritionally.**

Let's look at an analogy. Let's say you want to drive from New York to Philadelphia, a distance of 100 miles. Your gas tank is half-full, more than enough to get you there. What is the limiting factor of your trip? In other words, what is it that limits how long it takes you to get to Philadelphia?

If there's no traffic, the limiting factor is how fast you drive. If there is a lot of traffic, the limiting factor is how much traffic there is.

Now suppose someone told you, "Let me fill up your gas tank. That will get you there faster."

You would look at them as if they weren't running on all cylinders because clearly, if you had enough gas in the tank to start with, the amount of gas is not the limiting factor.

What does this have to do with nutrition?

Just because gasoline is involved in the trip from New York to Philadelphia does not mean that the *amount* of gasoline is the limiting factor. *Similarly, just because a certain nutrient is involved in the long sequence of chemical reactions does not mean that the* amount *of that nutrient is the limiting factor.*

You can have twelve times as much protein as you need and fifteen times as much carbohydrate and it would not change what comes out at the other end of the reaction one bit if the amount of protein or carbohydrate is not the limiting factor.

Certainly, if you didn't start with enough gasoline in the tank, *that* would become the limiting factor. Similarly, if you didn't start with enough protein, or carbohydrate, or this or that vitamin or mineral, *that* would become the limiting factor and could impair your performance.

But as long as you *do* have enough of the proper nutrients (an easy goal to achieve), more won't improve your performance.

The Handbook will often point out the limiting factor when talking about a nutritional practice. Correctly identifying limiting factors is essential to making accurate nutritional recommendations; *incorrectly* identifying them is the most common mistake behind erroneous ones.

■ For any series of reactions in the body (e.g. protein utilization, energy production), there is a *limiting factor.*

■ Common limiting factors include:

❑ one reaction in the series that proceeds more slowly than the rest of the reactions in the series

❑ a reaction that must be complete before other reactions can begin

❑ a nutrient that must be present in adequate quantities for one or more of the reactions to take place

■ Incorrectly identifying the limiting factor is the most common mistake behind erroneous nutritional recommendations.

■ Correctly identifying limiting factors can lead to substantial improvements in athletic nutrition.

❖   ❖   ❖

PART TWO

THE PHYSIOLOGY OF NUTRITION

This section covers individual nutrients, explaining what they are and what they do.

Bear in mind, however, that although the nutrients are discussed individually, each functions as an integral part of an incredibly complex system in which each nutrient is inseparably dependent on the others. It doesn't make sense to take one nutrient out of its "nutritional context" and make dietary changes based on the listed effects of that one nutrient. For example, although thiamine is involved in energy production, taking thiamine out of its "nutritional context" (taking more thiamine than you would otherwise get in a balanced athletic diet) will not make a major difference in athletic performance.

But we're getting ahead of ourselves. Before looking at the big picture, let's get down to the level of atoms, molecules, and cells, and take a close look at the physiology of nutrition.

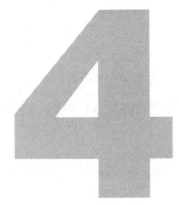

PROTEIN

THE BASIC FACTS

Every cell in your body contains protein. In fact, about three-quarters of the dry weight of most cells is protein. When most people think of protein, though, they usually only think of the most well-known protein, "muscle contractile protein." Actually, there are thousands of different kinds of proteins, and even "muscle contractile protein" is really eight different kinds of proteins.

Your body manufactures these thousands of different kinds of proteins by breaking down protein molecules from the food you eat, then reassembling and recombining their sub-parts in new ways. These sub-parts are called **amino acids**.

Amino acids are the building blocks from which protein molecules are constructed. There are twenty biologically important amino acids (see box). Each amino acid has a "nitrogen part" and a "carbon skeleton." The nitrogen part is the same for all twenty amino acids. The carbon part is different for every amino acid. A protein molecule is nothing more than a long string of these twenty amino acids connected end to end, much like beads in a necklace.

A Question of Order

How can proteins as different in structure and function as, say, **tropomyosin** (one of the eight muscle contractile proteins) and **insulin** (a hormone) be made from the same twenty amino acids? The key is the *sequence* of those amino acids. In the same way that the two words *interlaminations* and *internationalism* are

AMINO ACIDS

Alanine	Glycine	Proline
Arginine	Histidine	Serine
Asparagine	Isoleucine	Threonine
Aspartic acid	Leucine	Tryptophan
Cysteine	Lysine	Tyrosine
Glutamine	Methionine	Valine
Glutamic acid	Phenylalanine	

made from the same sixteen letters but have completely different meanings because of the *sequence* of those letters, so too are all the proteins in your body made from the same twenty amino acids but have completely different structures because of the *sequence* of those amino acids.

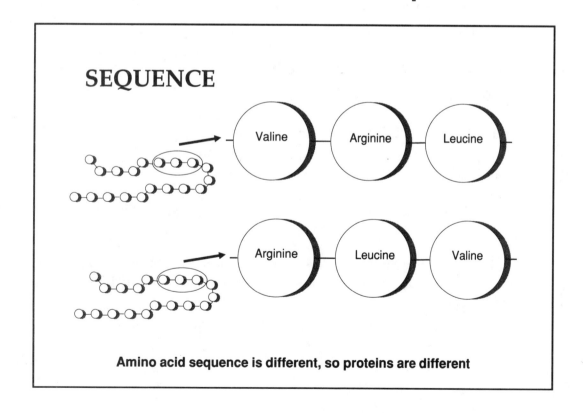

SEQUENCE

Amino acid sequence is different, so proteins are different

THE FOLLOWING ARE ALL PROTEINS...

All hormones (with the exception of steroid hormones)

insulin   growth hormone   glucagon   somatostatin

All enzymes

ptyalin   pepsin   trypsin   chymotrypsin   peptidases   proelastase procarboxypeptidases A and B   dehydrogenases   transaminases kinases   isomerases   carboxylases

Structural components

collagen   procollagen   keratin

Transport and storage molecules

hemoglobin   myoglobin   transferrin   ferritin

Immune components

antibodies

Cell communication components

hormone receptors   rhodopsin

Muscle contractile molecules

actin   myosin   troponin   tropomyosin   alpha-actinin beta-actinin   M protein   C protein

...and many, many more.

Some of these you've doubtless heard of, others are probably new to you. But you may not have realized before, they are all simply different kinds of proteins.

ESSENTIAL AMINO ACIDS

Isoleucine	Methionine	Tryptophan
Leucine	Phenylalanine	Valine
Lysine	Threonine	

Complete vs. Incomplete and Complementary Proteins

Of the twenty amino acids, eight are called **essential**. They are called this because your body cannot manufacture them in appreciable quantities. Since you can't make enough of them yourself, it is essential that you get them from your diet.

Foods that contain protein contain all or almost all of the same twenty amino acids, but in varying amounts and combinations. If a particular source of protein contains all eight essential amino acids, that protein is said to be *complete*. If a particular protein is deficient in any one of the eight amino acids, that protein is said to be *incomplete*.

Nature provides some complete protein sources—such as eggs, milk, fish, meat, and poultry—as well as incomplete protein sources—such as most grains and vegetables. Vegetable sources of protein are incomplete because they are lacking in one or more of the eight essential amino acids. For example,

EXAMPLES OF COMPLEMENTARY DIETARY PROTEINS

refried beans....with....corn tortillas
chili....with....cornbread
red beans....with....rice
lentils....with....rice
peanut butter......on......wheat bread
baked beans....with....wheat toast
bean.... and.....barley soup

corn is deficient in the essential amino acids **lysine** and **tryptophan**, and beans are deficient in the essential amino acid **methionine**.

Protein from incomplete sources can, however, be *combined* to form complete proteins. While corn is deficient in **lysine** and **tryptophan**, beans have plenty of **lysine** and **tryptophan**. And while beans are lacking in **methionine**, corn has plenty. So if you combine the two incomplete protein sources, corn and beans, you get a combination that is not deficient in any of the eight essential amino acids, and therefore is a complete protein. Incomplete proteins which can be be combined to form complete proteins are said to be *complementary*. (See box on previous page.)

WHAT HAPPENS WITH PROTEINS IN YOUR BODY

In Your Mouth

Chewing begins the digestive process by grinding your food into small particles. These small particles are mixed with saliva, which makes a soft, wet, easily swallowed mixture.

In Your Stomach

In your stomach, the gastric juice containing the enzyme **pepsin** starts to break down the protein—the long chains of amino acids—into shorter chains of amino acids.

In Your Intestines

Then, the partially-digested protein passes into your small intestine, where pancreatic juice containing certain enzymes further breaks down the protein into single amino acids and short chains a few amino acids long (**polypeptides**). Finally, a little farther along in your small intestine, another group of enzymes called **peptidases** break down the polypeptides into single amino acids, and chains two or three amino acids long (**dipeptides** and **tripeptides**, respectively). The single amino acids, dipeptides, and tripeptides are ready to be absorbed into your bloodstream.

PROTEIN BREAKDOWN IN THE SMALL INTESTINE

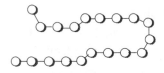

Protein

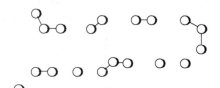

STEP 2: Polypeptides broken down into *mono-*, *di-*, and *tripeptides*

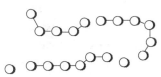

STEP 1: Protein broken down into *polypeptides* (short chains of amino acids) and single amino acids

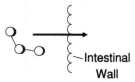

STEP 3: Peptides absorbed

In Your Blood

And absorbed they are. These single amino acids, dipeptides, and tripeptides pass through the intestinal walls and enter your bloodstream, which transports them to the liver. From there one of four things happens: a given amino acid can...

- re-enter the bloodstream and continue on to the rest of the body
- be converted into a different amino acid
- be used as is to make one kind of protein or another
- be broken down further.

By no means do all the amino acids you eat get incorporated into protein. Which of the four fates a given amino acid will undergo depends on the demands of your body at the time you eat the protein.

Your body needs a certain amount of protein every day, about 0.8 gm/kg/day, for normal growth, repair, and maintenance. Athletes, including bodybuilders, need slightly more—about 1.0 gm/kg/day (80 grams per day for a 176-pound athlete);

some estimates go as high as 1.5 gm/kg/day. The average American intake is two to three times that. Bodybuilders often eat 7 gm/kg/day or more—far in excess of what their bodies need or can use.

As an athlete, if you don't eat your 1.0 to 1.5 gm/kg every day, you won't have enough raw materials with which to manufacture new proteins for normal daily growth, repair, and maintenance. Your body will have to turn to internal sources, such as your liver and muscle, for amino acids. This may mean some loss of muscle mass and muscle strength.

Even if you **do** eat your 1.0 to 1.5 gm/kg of protein every day, if it's not complete protein or complementary proteins you won't be able to manufacture new proteins for normal daily growth, repair, and maintenance. It's like trying to spell but missing the vowels—it doesn't matter how many consonants you have, if you don't have any vowels you can't spell anything. Similarly, if your body doesn't have lysine or tryptophan or any other of the eight essential amino acids, it can't build proteins, no matter how many of the non-essential amino acids are about. Again, your body will have to turn to internal sources, such as your liver and muscle, for amino acids. Again, this may mean some loss of muscle mass and muscle strength.

Now let's say you eat an average American protein intake of 3 gm/kg/day, and let's say the protein you are eating is complete (as is true for people who get their protein from meat). During the course of a normal day, your body takes about 1.0 to 1.5 gm/kg of amino acids from the 3 gm/kg of proteins you eat and manufactures new proteins from them.

What happens to the amino acids in the 1.5 to 2.0 gm/kg that *didn't* get incorporated into proteins? We know that they can have only one of three other fates: re-entering the blood stream and travelling on to other cells, being converted into other amino acids, or being broken down further.

All three of these fates occur, but the first two simply keep the amino acids in circulation for a while. Eventually they must fall to the third fate, that of being broken down further.

When an amino acid is broken down further, it is no longer an amino acid. Most of the nitrogen part gets converted into urea and excreted in the urine. Most of the carbon part—the *carbon skeleton*—gets stored as fat.

None of the excess protein is converted into muscle protein or in any way enhances athletic performance.

BIO-AVAILABILITY, FREE-FORM AMINO ACIDS, PROTEIN EFFICIENCY RATIO

Bioavailability

Bioavailability refers to the degree to which a nutrient is accessible for biologic use by the human body. When talking about proteins, it refers to how easily the protein is broken down into its component amino acids. Almost all sources of dietary protein have high bioavailability. Those that have low bioavailability—the proteins in hair, fingernails, feathers, hoofs, horns, scales—don't usually show up in normal diets.

When a protein supplement boasts of "high bioavailability," the manufacturers are trying to buffalo you into thinking that somehow their protein is more readily absorbed than others. In fact, what it means is that the protein source for their supplement was not hair, fingernails, feathers, hoofs, horns, or scales.

Free-Form Amino Acids

With that in mind, what about **free-form** or **purified** or **crystalline amino acids**? In this case, someone has gone to the trouble of having a lab do the digestion for you. Instead of getting your amino acids from food, in the long chains we call proteins, you get your amino acids already broken down into individual amino acids or short chains two or three amino acids long.

The manufacturers of these products claim that the amino acids in pre-digested proteins (which is what these supplements are) are more readily absorbed than amino acids from normal food. But again, unless your dietary protein source is hair, fingernails, feathers, hoofs, horns, or scales, your protein source already **has** high bioavailability. You don't gain anything by eating free-form amino acids.

Protein Efficiency Ratios

Protein efficiency ratio *(P.E.R.)* refers to the ratios of essential amino acids in protein-rich foods. You need all eight in your diet, but not all in the same quantities. Manufacturers of protein supplements have capitalized on this fact, by making protein supplements that provide essential amino acid ratios close to the ratios that your body needs. Sounds like a great idea.

The only people for whom protein efficiency ratios have any real meaning are those whose protein intakes border on deficiency (for example, strict vegetarians that pay no attention to complementary proteins). If they are going to eat the absolute minimum amount of protein necessary to be healthy, it makes sense for them to eat the essential amino acids in the proper proportions. For the rest of us, however, protein deficiency is not a concern, and protein efficiency ratios are meaningless.

Protein as Fuel

Protein is also used as fuel for energy, to a much greater extent than had been previously thought. After four hours of continuous exercise, up to forty-five percent of the fuel for energy can come from protein sources, mostly muscle. Although, as we shall see, carbohydrates and fat should be your primary energy sources, when short of carbohydrates your body obtains progressively higher percentages of total energy from protein.

However, this is your body's emergency measure, and should be minimized. Protein used as fuel cannot be used for cell repair or replacement, for muscle contraction, or for any of the important functions mentioned above. Athletes involved in heavy endurance training (who are the only ones who really need to concern themselves with this problem) can minimize use of protein as fuel for energy by maintaining a high intake of carbohydrates.

Too Much

Your cells are involved in a constant cycle of breakdown and rebuilding. Your body constantly requires new *incoming* protein to replace the *outgoing* amino acids in the cells. Ideally, your diet should provide just enough amino acids to replace the proteins that have broken down.

If you consume much more protein than you need—as most people in the United States do—the excess amino acids will be broken down, with the carbon skeletons stored as fat and the nitrogen part excreted as urea. All this excess urea can significantly strain your liver and kidneys.

Too Little

On the flip side, since protein is required in every cell for so many different processes, protein deficiency hurts the entire body. Serious protein deficiency, which is rare in the United States, is called **kwashiorkor**, and is characterized by stunted growth, malnutrition, and sometimes death. Even mild shortages of protein can impair your body's rebuilding processes and disrupt important regulatory functions.

Thus, although it is unlikely that you consume too little protein, it is worth figuring it out to be sure. And if you find you are consuming too much protein and decide to cut down, you must be sure to continue getting enough to meet your needs.

People—such as bodybuilders—who do hard physical work, generally do *not* need greatly increased amounts of protein. Rather, they need only small increases in protein, but substantial increases in *calories*.

In contrast, infants, children, teenagers, pregnant women, and lactating mothers *do* need substantially more protein. Older people generally require *less* protein; however, because their bodies may not use protein as efficiently as in younger years, older people may have to eat more protein to satisfy their bodies' needs.

That brings us to the numbers. How much of your diet should consist of protein? In terms of calories, the answer is about ten to fifteen percent. So if your energy requirement is, say, 3000 calories per day (we'll figure it out in Chapter 18), you should be getting between 300 and 450 of those calories from protein.

■ There are thousands of different kinds of proteins in the body; *muscle proteins* are just eight of those.

■ Proteins are made up of long strings of smaller units called *amino acids*.

❑ The *sequence* of the amino acids in the long string is what makes one protein different from another.

❑ There are twenty biologically important amino acids. Eight are called *essential* because your body cannot manufacture them; you must get them in the food you eat.

❑ Just as you can't spell anything unless the vowels are present, your body can't manufacture all the different kinds of proteins it needs unless the essential amino acids are present.

❑ Protein in foods containing all eight essential amino acids is called *complete* protein.

❑ Protein in foods that don't contain all eight essential amino acids is called *incomplete* protein.

❑ Pairs of protein sources which are incomplete individually but complete when combined are called *complementary* proteins.

■ Most people—bodybuilders and other athletes included—eat much more protein than they need for optimum performance and maximum muscle growth.

  ❑ The average person requires 0.5 to 0.8 grams of protein per kilogram of bodyweight per day.

  ❑ Bodybuilders and other athletes require slightly more, about 1.0 to 1.5 grams per kilogram of bodyweight per day.

  ❑ The average person in the U.S. gets two to three grams per kilogram of bodyweight per day—*twice as much as even the bodybuilder needs*.

■ Eating too much protein is bad for your health, and can hurt your athletic performance.

❖   ❖   ❖

CARBOHYDRATES

THE BASIC FACTS

There are three kinds of carbohydrates: **monosaccharides**, **disaccharides**, and **polysaccharides**. Monosaccharides and disaccharides are also called **simple sugars**. Polysaccharides are also called **complex carbohydrates**.

Simple Sugars

Monosaccharides are the simplest carbohydrates, consisting only of single molecules of sugar (*mono* = one, *saccharide* = sugar). The two most common monosaccharides are **fructose** (called *fruit sugar*, because it occurs naturally in many fruits), and **glucose** (called *blood sugar*, because it is found in the blood).

   Disaccharides are carbohydrates made of two single molecules of sugar (two monosaccharides) linked together (*di* = two). The most common disaccharides are **sucrose**, **lactose**, and **maltose**. Sucrose (ordinary table sugar) is a disaccharide made by linking together the monosaccharides fructose and glucose. **Lactose** (called *milk sugar*, because it is naturally present in milk), is a disaccharide made by linking together the monosaccharides galactose and glucose. **Maltose** (made from the breakdown of starch in the malting of barley, and most commonly found in sprouted grains) is a disaccharide made by linking together two molecules of glucose.

Polysaccharides are carbohydrates made of many single molecules of sugar (monosaccharides) linked together into long branched chains (*poly* = many). Polysaccharides exist in three forms: **starch**, **glycogen**, and **cellulose**.

Starch is the form in which plants store carbohydrates. It is commonly found in potatoes, grains, and other vegetable sources.

Glycogen is the form in which animals store carbohydrates. When you eat carbohydrates, some of the monosaccharides you absorb into your bloodstream get stored in your liver and muscles as glycogen.

Cellulose is a carbohydrate, but unlike starch and glycogen it is not a storage carbohydrate. It is a **structural carbohydrate**, an integral part of the physical structure of most plants.

Monosaccharides can be linked together in many different ways, and it is the *way* they are linked together that makes the polysaccharide starch, glycogen, or cellulose. The monosaccharides in cellulose are linked together in such a way that they can't be broken apart by your digestive enzymes. This makes cellulose indigestible, and is why humans can't digest grass or trees.

So all carbohydrates—from the sugar in your sugar bowl to the cellulose in sawdust—are made from single molecules of sugar (monosaccharides) linked together in different ways.

Complex Carbohydrates

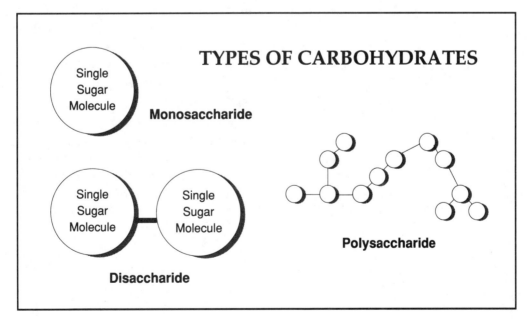

TYPES OF CARBOHYDRATES

Single Sugar Molecule — Monosaccharide

Single Sugar Molecule — Single Sugar Molecule — Disaccharide

Polysaccharide

Food Processing

In your small intestine, all digestible polysaccharides are broken down into the monosaccharides glucose, fructose, and galactose. (The indigestible polysaccharides pass on to the large intestine.) Only in the form of monosaccharides can carbohydrates pass through the intestinal wall into your bloodstream. Once in your bloodstream, they are transported to the **liver**.

Blood Sugar

Glucose is the most common monosaccharide, and once absorbed through the intestinal wall its concentration can be measured in the bloodstream. This concentration is called the **blood sugar** level. Your blood sugar level must remain within certain boundaries. Through a whole host of complex homeostatic mechanisms, your body monitors and adjusts your blood sugar level to keep it within those boundaries. When the level of glucose in your blood gets too high, your body sends the hormone **insulin** into your bloodstream to bring your glucose level down (in the same way a person with **diabetes mellitus** takes insulin to bring blood sugar down; **diabetes mellitus** is, in fact, a disorder of carbohydrate regulation). When the level of glucose in your blood gets too low, your body sends **glucagon** into your bloodstream to bring your glucose level up.

Carbohydrates— the Athlete's Energy Fuel

Regardless of a carbohydrate's original form—monosaccharide, disaccharide, or polysaccharide—all carbohydrates are monosaccharides (mostly glucose) when they reach your liver. Your liver stores some of the glucose as *glycogen*, and sends the rest back into your bloodstream to provide immediate energy for the rest of your body, to be stored in the muscles as glycogen, or to be converted into fat.

When your muscles need energy, they use the glucose floating around in your blood first. This causes your blood sugar level to fall, which causes glucagon to be released. Glucagon causes stored glycogen to be converted back into glucose, restoring your blood sugar level to normal and providing a steady supply of fuel.

Carbohydrates do much more than just supply energy. Carbohydrates help your body utilize proteins and fats properly (another reason why the *balance* of nutrients is so important). A proper intake of carbohydrates has a "protein sparing" effect—it allows your body to burn glucose for energy instead of burning muscle protein. Carbohydrates are also important in the structure of skin, cartilage, tendons, cell membranes, genetic material, intercellular "glue," and many other tissue components.

Cellulose, an indigestible carbohydrate, is one type of **fiber** (fiber is discussed in detail in Chapter 9). Fiber has been receiving increasing attention for its potential role in disease prevention.

The issue of simple versus complex carbohydrates is complicated.

It is an oversimplification to state categorically, *All simple carbohydrates are bad*. Simple carbohydrates, such as fructose, are present in high concentrations in fruit, and nutritionists widely recommend increased intake of fresh fruit. The problem is that little of the simple carbohydrates in the American diet are from fruit. The average American consumes over a quarter-pound of table sugar a day, most of it in the form of soft drinks, candy, cookies, and pre-sweetened cereals. These foods provide lots of calories but are of little nutritional value besides that. In addition, excess sugar intake is thought to be involved somehow with diabetes, obesity, and coronary artery disease. (Sugar is examined in depth in Chapter 9.)

Complex carbohydrates, on the other hand, tend to be found in foods that are also rich in vitamins, minerals, and fiber such as whole wheat products, potatoes, and dried beans and peas. On the whole, they are a better nutritional choice.

Which get into your bloodstream faster, simple or complex carbohydrates? For years it was thought that simple carbohydrates got into your bloodstream faster, because they didn't have to go through the digestive process. In recent studies, however, carbohydrate from some simple-carbohydrate foods has been shown to be absorbed more slowly than carbohydrate from some complex-carbohydrate foods. For example, the carbohydrate in a candy bar has been shown to be absorbed *more*

WHAT CARBOHYDRATE DOES FOR YOU

Simple vs. Complex

The Glycemic Index

slowly than carbohydrate from whole wheat bread. The same studies also reported that the simple carbohydrates in fruit were absorbed even more slowly than the simple carbohydrates in the candy bar.

These comparisons are only meaningful when considering differences in absorption time for individual foods (a candy bar eaten alone versus a potato eaten alone, for example). When foods are eaten together, as they are during a meal, a host of factors affect absorption time, rendering these comparisons irrelevant.

This has not stopped a few nutritional writers from drawing sweeping conclusions from the new data. Some have even said you are more likely to gain weight by including potatoes in your diet than by including ice cream—or, more generally, that you are more likely to gain weight eating foods with a high **glycemic index** (indicating faster absorption) than eating foods with a low glycemic index.

This overlooks the simple fact that the overriding factor affecting weight control is calories, not absorption time. A pint of ice cream, containing about 900 calories, is still more likely to make you gain weight than an equivalent volume of russet potatoes, containing about 180 calories, even though the potatoes have a higher glycemic index.

The glycemic index is important to the athlete in selecting the best pre- and during-competition snacks, a subject discussed in Chapter 20.

How Much Carbohydrate?

Because your body constantly uses glucose for fuel, you must replenish your supplies regularly. If you eat too little carbohydrate, muscle and liver glycogen stores are quickly depleted, impairing both aerobic and anaerobic performance.

How much of your diet should consist of carbohydrates? The average person should be getting from fifty-five to sixty percent of all calories from carbohydrates, with no more than about ten percent of total calories coming from simple carbohydrates. For you, as an athlete, the numbers are slightly higher—sixty to sixty-five percent of all calories. If you regularly participate in endurance events, the numbers are higher still—sixty-five to seventy percent of all calories from carbohydrates, with no more than ten percent from simple carbohydrates.

■ All carbohydrates—from the sugar in your sugar bowl to the cellulose in sawdust—are made from single molecules of sugar linked together in different ways.

■ There are three kinds of carbohydrates:

❑ *Monosaccharides,* which are single sugar molecules (Examples: fructose, glucose)

❑ *Disaccharides,* which consist of two monosaccharides linked together (Examples: sucrose, lactose)

❑ *Polysaccharides,* which consist of three or more monosaccharides linked together

■ Monosaccharides and disaccharides are also called *simple sugars.* Polysaccharides are also called *complex carbohydrates.*

■ Most foods containing complex carbohydrates have a higher nutritional value than foods containing primarily simple sugars.

■ Contrary to the long-held belief that complex carbohydrates are absorbed more slowly than simple sugars, current research indicates the relationship between carbohydrate complexity and absorption time is not that simple. Some complex carbohydrates are absorbed more quickly than some simple sugars.

- There are three kinds of polysaccharides: *starch, glycogen, and cellulose.*

- All digestible carbohydrates you eat are broken down into monosaccharides. Only as monosaccharides can carbohydrates be absorbed through the wall of the small intestine into your bloodstream.

- Your body stores carbohydrate in your liver and muscles as *glycogen.*

- Carbohydrate circulates in your blood in the form of glucose. When enough circulating glucose is taken up by your muscles for use in energy production, glycogen from the liver is converted into glucose and sent out into the blood to maintain your *blood sugar level* within narrow boundaries.

- Guideline for optimum athletic performance:

  ❑ The majority of your dietary calories should come from complex carbohydrates. Specifically...

  ❑ For the average person, 55-60% of calories from carbs, no more than 10% from simple sugars

  ❑ For the athlete, 60-65% of calories from carbs, no more than 10% from simple sugars

  ❑ For the endurance athlete, 65-70% of calories from carbs, no more than 5% from simple sugars

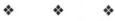

FATS

THE BASIC FACTS

People often don't think of fats and oils as nutrients at all, let alone as indispensable ones. Yet in spite of their unglamorous image, fats and oils are essential to the proper functioning of the body. In this chapter, we'll take a look at what fat is, how your body handles it, and what it does for you.

Saturated versus Unsaturated

A fat molecule is made of three parallel **fatty acid** chains linked at one end to a glycerine molecule. The whole molecule looks a lot like the business end of a fork.

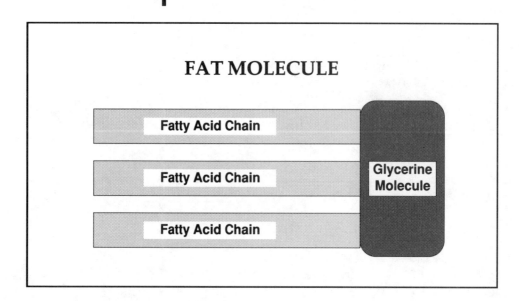

FAT MOLECULE

Fatty Acid Chain

Fatty Acid Chain

Fatty Acid Chain

Glycerine Molecule

Each of the three individual fatty acid chains falls into one of two categories: **saturated** or **unsaturated**.

The difference between the two is a matter of hydrogen atoms. Hydrogen atoms attach to a fatty acid chain in pairs. There are a number of places on the fatty acid chain where pairs of hydrogen atoms can attach. If all the places on the fatty acid chain where pairs of hydrogen atoms can attach have hydrogen atoms attached to them, the chain is *saturated* with hydrogens and is referred to as a **saturated fat**. Butter is an example of a saturated fat. On the other hand, if not all the places hydrogen atoms can attach have pairs of hydrogen atoms attached, the chain is *not* saturated with hydrogens, and is called an **unsaturated fat**.

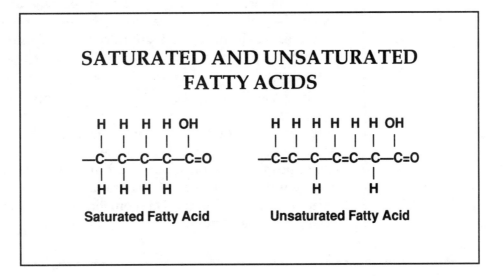

SATURATED AND UNSATURATED FATTY ACIDS

Saturated Fatty Acid

Unsaturated Fatty Acid

Monounsaturated versus Polyunsaturated

Just as fatty acids can be divided into saturated and unsaturated, the category of unsaturated fatty acids can further be divided into two other categories. Depending on how close an unsaturated fatty acid chain is to being saturated, it's called either *monounsaturated* or *polyunsaturated*. As you might guess, a fatty acid only one pair of hydrogens short of being saturated is called **monounsaturated** (*mono* = one).

Examples of monounsaturated fats are olive, peanut and avocado oils.

A fatty acid more than one pair of hydrogens short of being saturated is called **polyunsaturated** (*poly* = many). Examples— corn, safflower, and soybean oils.

In general, saturated fats tend to raise the level of cholesterol in your blood, increasing the risk of atherosclerotic coronary artery disease (hardening of the arteries), while polyunsaturated fats tend to *lower* blood cholesterol, decreasing the risk of atherosclerotic coronary artery disease. Monounsaturated fats, once thought to have no effect on blood cholesterol, have now been shown to lower cholesterol as much as, or perhaps more than, polyunsaturated fats.

Dozens of different fatty acids are present in our foods. All natural sources of fat contain both saturated and unsaturated fatty acids. However, meats and other animal proteins contain primarily saturated fatty acids, while vegetable sources contain larger proportions of unsaturated fatty acids.

For example, butter has about sixty-six percent saturated fats, thirty-one percent monounsaturates, and three percent polyunsaturates. Soybean oil has about fifteen percent saturated fats, twenty-five percent monounsaturates, and sixty percent polyunsaturates.

What's the difference between a fat and an oil? They are both collections of fat molecules, but a fat is solid at room temperature, and an oil is liquid at room temperature. They have the same number of calories. What makes one collection of fat molecules solid at room temperature and another liquid at room temperature is the degree of saturation. The more saturated the fat, the more solid at room temperature; the less saturated, the more runny.

BUYER BEWARE!

Ever see the phrase *hydrogenated vegetable oil* on an ingredient list and wonder what it meant? It means that the product you are eating started with an unsaturated vegetable oil (more healthful) that the processor combined with extra hydrogen, making the unsaturated oil more saturated (less healthful).

Saturated fats have a longer shelf life than unsaturated fats, and it's cheaper to start with an unsaturated fat (such as soybean oil) and hydrogenate it than to use a saturated fat (such as butter).

Butter, lard, and vegetable shortening, all solid at room temperature, are highly saturated. Olive, peanut, and avocado oils, liquid at room temperature, are monounsaturated. Corn, sunflower, and soybean oils, also liquid at room temperature but runnier than olive, peanut, or avocado oils, are polyunsaturated.

Essential Fatty Acids

Regardless of which fat sources you use, your body is capable of manufacturing *almost* all of the many different fatty acids it needs from what you give it. But, as with amino acids, there are a few fatty acids your body must have but *cannot* manufacture. These are called the **essential** fatty acids, and you must consume them in your diet.

There are two: **linoleic acid** and **linolenic acid**. Both are unsaturated—**your body does not require any saturated fats.**

Where do you get linoleic and linolenic acids? Most plants are excellent sources of both.

WHAT HAPPENS WITH FATS IN THE BODY

In Your Mouth

Fats and oils enter your mouth as three parts fatty acid and one part glycerine. (Another word for fat molecule is **triglyceride**—three [*tri* = three] fatty acids for every glycerine.) Unlike carbohydrates, fats do not begin breaking down in your mouth.

In Your Stomach

They go on to your stomach, where they mix with proteins and carbohydrates to form a sludgy mass called **chyme**.

In Your Small Intestine

The chyme passes from your stomach into your small intestine, where it is **emulsified**—broken down into small fat globules—by **bile**, a product of your liver and gall bladder. This emulsification process prepares the fats to be acted upon by an enzyme called **pancreatic lipase**.

Pancreatic lipase separates two of the three fatty acids from the glycerine in each fat molecule, leaving two fatty acids and a **monoglyceride**. These fatty acid and monoglyceride molecules then get absorbed through the intestinal walls, are reassembled into fat molecules (triglycerides), enter your lymphatic system, and eventually reach your bloodstream.

In Your Blood

Now, oil and water don't mix. So how does a fat molecule, essentially an oil, move through the blood, which is mostly water? It travels with the aid of some special protein molecules, called **apoproteins**, in special transport carriers, called **lipoproteins**.

When the newly-absorbed fat molecule is leaving your intestines, it gathers together with a lot of other fat molecules, some cholesterol, and some apoprotein molecules and forms a lipoprotein called a **chylomicron**. Chylomicrons are responsible for transporting fat molecules and cholesterol to fat cells and your liver.

Other types of lipoproteins, **very low density lipoproteins (VLDL's)**, **low density lipoproteins (LDL's)**, and **high density lipoproteins (HDL's)** will be discussed in the chapter on cholesterol (Chapter 9).

What Fats Do For You

Fat does much more than just bring a lot of calories into your body. Fat:

- protects your internal organs from injury by forming a natural protective layer over them
- *insulates*—it helps keep you warm by guarding against excessive loss of body heat when the outside temperature goes down
- serves as a source of energy. Fat is your primary source of energy at rest, and the source of about 50% of the energy for light and moderate exercise. For prolonged moderate exercise, fat provides over 80% of the energy.
- is your primary long-term storehouse for energy
- is necessary for absorption of fat-soluble nutrients— vitamins A, D, E, and K.

How Much Fat?

As with protein and carbohydrates, you need a certain amount of fat in your daily diet. Getting enough is seldom a problem, though. Fat tastes good. In fact, fat is the primary difference between supermarket ice cream and "gourmet" ice cream—gourmet ice cream contains about sixty percent more!

Most Americans consume far too much fat. Translated into excess body fat, this not only interferes with athletic performance, it is dangerous to your health. Fat increases your risk of heart disease, and may be linked to certain kinds of cancer.

Once again, that brings us to the numbers. How much of your diet should consist of fat?

You must have a minimum of one to two percent of your calories from fat, to get the essential linoleic and linolenic acids you need every day, and to absorb the necessary fat-soluble vitamins.

The average American gets forty-two percent of his or her calories from fat, so there is little concern about not getting enough. Ideally, less than twenty percent of your calories should be from fat. Since this limit is a little hard to adhere to, given the current assortment of food preferences of the American public, the Senate Select Committee on Nutrition recommends a fat intake of thirty percent of all calories, with no more than ten percent coming from saturated fats.

Let's put that another way. If your energy requirement is 3000 calories per day, you should be getting between 600 and 900 of those calories from fats. Less than ten percent of your total calories—300, in this example—should come from saturated fats. The rest of your fat calories should come from monounsaturated and polyunsaturated fats.

- ■ Fat molecules are made up of simpler units called *fatty acids*

- ■ Fatty acids can be either *saturated* or *unsaturated*

- ■ Unsaturated fatty acids can be either *mono*unsaturated and *poly*unsaturated.

- The more liquid (runny) the fat or oil, the more unsaturated it is.

- Saturated fat intake *increases* blood cholesterol and poses a serious health risk.

- Unsaturated fat intake *decreases* blood cholesterol, decreasing risk of heart and circulatory disease.

- Fat is an essential part of your diet.

  - ❏ Fat protects your internal organs, keeps you warm, is necessary for absorption of fat-soluble vitamins A, D, E, and K, and serves as a source of energy.

- Guidelines for Optimum Athletic Nutrition:

  - ❏ You must have a small amount of fat in your diet—at least 1 to 2% of your daily caloric intake.

  - ❏ You should get no more than 30% of your daily calories from fats.

  - ❏ No more than 10% of those calories should be from saturated fats.

❖   ❖   ❖

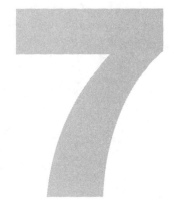

VITAMINS

Vitamins are organic chemicals essential to normal human metabolism. They occur in tiny amounts in foods. Although humans do not require large doses of vitamins, they must consume enough to meet minimum requirements, or disease results.

There are currently thirteen compounds officially recognized as vitamins: **A** (retinol), **B1** (thiamine), **B2** (riboflavin), **B3** (niacin), **B6** (pyridoxine), **B12** (cyanocobalamin), **folic acid**, **biotin**, **pantothenic acid**, **C**, **D**, **E**, and **K**.

There are also a number of chemicals, including **inositol**, **choline**, **pangamic acid** ("vitamin B15"), and **laetrile** ("vitamin B17") which are not vitamins at all but are sometimes mistakenly called so.

Each of the recognized vitamins is essential in dozens of chemical reactions occurring in the body. Lack of any vitamin impairs or halts the specific reactions for which it is required, and produces specific deficiency symptoms.

Sufficient amounts of all the vitamins are necessary for the body's chemical reactions to run at top efficiency; therefore, sufficient amounts of all the vitamins are necessary for peak performance. Many of the vitamins can be harmful in excess dosages, however, so it is important to ensure adequate vitamin intake without going overboard.

The vitamins are classified into two groups: **water-soluble** (those which dissolve in water but not in fat) and **fat-soluble** (those which dissolve in fat but not in water).

WATER-SOLUBLE VITAMINS

The water-soluble vitamins are **B1, B2, B3, B6, B12, folic acid, biotin**, and **pantothenic acid** (collectively known as the **B-complex**), and **vitamin C**.

For the most part, they are not stored in any appreciable amounts (vitamin B12 is an exception). This means adequate quantities of the B-complex and vitamin C need to be eaten every day. They can also be excreted in the urine, which means excess amounts are cleared from the body quickly (in an attempt to return to homeostatic levels).

The water-soluble vitamins may be easily destroyed by cooking, leeched out in cooking water, or broken down as food loses freshness. For this reason, fruits and vegetables are best served raw or lightly steamed, and eaten soon after purchase.

B1 (Thiamine)

B1, RDA: 1.4-1.5 mg (male), 1.0-1.1 mg (female)

Good sources: pork, organ meats, whole grains and enriched cereals, peas, beans.

Carbohydrates are eventually oxidized into carbon dioxide and water. Thiamine participates in this energy-releasing process by helping to release the carbon dioxide. The greater your caloric intake, the more thiamine you need.

A severe deficiency of thiamine causes *beriberi*, which is characterized by mental confusion, muscle weakness, heart problems, and leg cramps.

Studies have shown that a mild thiamine deficiency can cause decreased aerobic performance, slower reaction time, decreased strength, decreased physical efficiency, fatigue, "lack of pep," and increased leg pain during work. These findings were reversed with thiamine replacement. **However, further thiamine supplementation beyond recommended levels produced no further improvement in physical performance.**

Excessive thiamine is not known to cause any problems.

B2 (Riboflavin)

B2, RDA: 1.6-1.7 mg (male), 1.2-1.3 mg (female)

Good sources: liver, milk, meat, dark green vegetables, eggs, whole grains and enriched cereals, peas, beans.

Riboflavin is important in breaking down and releasing energy from fatty acids, amino acids, and carbohydrates. The greater your protein intake, the more riboflavin you need.

A deficiency of riboflavin causes specific skin problems (*seborrheic dermatitis* of the face), cracks at the corners of the mouth, and sensitivity of the eyes to light. Although riboflavin is necessary for energy production, riboflavin deficiency has not been shown to have any detrimental effect on strength or endurance.

Excessive riboflavin is not known to cause any problems.

B3 (Niacin)

B3, RDA: 18-19 mg (male), 13-14 mg (female)

Good sources: liver, poultry, meat, tuna, eggs, whole grains and enriched cereals, beans, nuts. Niacin can be formed from the amino acid **tryptophan**.

Niacin, along with thiamine and riboflavin, is important in energy production. The greater your caloric intake, the more niacin you need.

A severe deficiency of niacin causes *pellegra*, which is characterized by skin lesions, diarrhea, and mental problems.

Excess niacin causes flushing, burning, and tingling around the neck, face, and hands, and increases the risk of ulcer and gout.

Several experiments have been done looking into the effects of supplemental niacin on endurance. It appears niacin slows release of free fatty acids from fat during both exercise and rest, decreasing the availability of free fatty acids as a fuel for energy production. This causes a greater reliance on glycogen stores for fuel, which may deplete these stores earlier and compromise performance. Theoretically, then, niacin supplementation could compromise performance; experimentally, however, niacin supplementation has not been shown to worsen aerobic performance.

On the other hand, while not worsening performance, niacin supplementation has been shown to alter the *perception* of exercise: experimental subjects perceived exercise after niacin to be heavier and more fatiguing than identical exercise after placebo.

B6, RDA: 2.2 mg (male), 2.0 mg (female)

Good sources: liver, meat, whole grain cereals, green leafy vegetables, nuts.

Vitamin B6 is important in breaking down amino acids, in forming one amino acid from another, in the production of hemoglobin and myoglobin, and in breaking down glycogen into glucose. The greater your protein intake, the more vitamin B6 you need.

A deficiency of vitamin B6 causes irritability, convulsions, muscular twitching, skin problems, cracks at the corners of the mouth, kidney stones, dizziness, nausea, anemia. Most pregnant women are deficient in vitamin B6, and oral contraceptives may cause a mild deficiency.

Some researchers have speculated that since vitamin B6 is important in releasing glucose from glycogen, B6 supplementation may cause a more-rapid depletion of glycogen stores during exercise following a low-carbohydrate diet. In this instance, B6 supplementation would be expected to *worsen* aerobic performance. In fact, B6 supplementation has not been shown to have any effect on aerobic performance.

Excessive vitamin B6 may cause a dependency on a high doses, leading to a vitamin B6 deficiency when the excess is withdrawn.

B12, RDA: 0.003 mg (male), 0.003 mg (female)

Good sources: liver, milk, meat, eggs, kidneys. Vitamin B12 is only found in foods of animal origin.

Vitamin B12 is important in proper formation of red blood cells and proper functioning of the nervous system.

A deficiency of vitamin B12 causes a type of anemia called **pernicious anemia**, which is characterized by fatigue, pale skin, and numbness and tingling that may progress to arm and leg weakness. Since vitamin B12 is only found in foods of animal origin, strict vegetarians are at risk of developing pernicious anemia. However, the liver stores relatively large amounts of vitamin B12, and very little is needed, so it may take years for a deficiency to show up with symptoms.

Vitamin B12 supplementation is common among athletes, with some receiving 1 gram injections an hour before competition. **However, studies have consistently failed to demon-**

**B6
(Pyridoxal
Phosphate)**

**B12
(Cyanocobalamin)**

strate any improvement in strength or endurance with B12 supplementation.

Excessive vitamin B12 is not known to cause any problems.

Folic acid

Folic Acid, RDA: 0.4 mg (male), 0.4 mg (female)

Good sources: liver and kidney, dark-green leafy vegetables, whole wheat products, peas, beans.

Folic acid is important in the formation of amino acids, genetic material, and hemoglobin.

A deficiency of folic acid causes a type of anemia called **megaloblastic anemia**, which is characterized by fatigue, abnormally large red blood cells, and diarrhea.

No research has been done investigating the effects of folic acid supplementation on physical performance.

Excessive folic acid is not known to cause any problems.

Biotin

Biotin, RDA: 0.10-0.20 mg (male), 0.10-0.20 mg (female)

Good sources: liver and kidneys, dark-green leafy vegetables, peas, beans, egg yolks. Biotin is also made by intestinal bacteria.

Biotin is important in the formation of fatty acids, amino acids, and glycogen.

A deficiency of biotin causes fatigue, depression, nausea, dermatitis, and muscular pains. Because the body has a dual supply of biotin (you get it both from food and from intestinal bacteria), deficiencies are rare. However, raw egg white has a substance, **avidin,** which binds to biotin in the intestinal tract and prevents its absorption, so eating large amounts of raw egg white conceivably could cause a biotin deficiency. Cooking destroys avidin, so cooked egg white has no effect on biotin.

No research has been done investigating the effects of biotin supplementation on physical performance.

Excessive biotin is not known to cause any problems.

Pantothenic acid

Pantothenic Acid, RDA: 4-7 mg (male), 4-7 mg (female)

Good sources: liver and kidneys, dark-green leafy vegetables, peas, beans, eggs. Pantothenic acid is found in all foods.

Pantothenic acid is a necessary component in Coenzyme A (CoA), which plays a central role in the production of energy from glucose and fatty acids.

A deficiency of pantothenic acid causes fatigue, sleep disturbances, impaired coordination, nausea and vomiting. Because pantothenic acid is found in all foods, deficiencies are quite rare.

No research has been done investigating the effects of pantothenic acid supplementation on physical performance.

Excessive pantothenic acid is not known to cause any problems.

Vitamin C, RDA: 60 mg (male), 60 mg (female)

Good sources: citrus fruits, tomatoes, green peppers, strawberries, potatoes, dark-green leafy vegetables. Vitamin C is largely destroyed by cooking.

Vitamin C is important in the formation of collagen, cartilage, bone, and teeth, and the *fight or flight* hormone **epinephrine** (also called **adrenaline**). It also protects other vitamins from inactivation, and participates in immune defenses. It is claimed by some to be protective against colds, viruses, and certain types of cancer when taken in large doses; research on these claims is not conclusive.

A deficiency of vitamin C causes **scurvy**, a disease characterized by degeneration of skin, teeth, blood vessels, muscles, easy bruising and bleeding, and poor healing.

In people with mild deficiencies, vitamin C supplementation improves physical performance. In most well-controlled studies, supplementation to beyond the RDA has failed to produce further improvements in either aerobic or anaerobic performance.

It has been claimed that supplemental vitamin C can reduce severity and recovery time associated with athletic injuries. However, placebo-controlled trials have failed to support this.

Excessive vitamin C may cause kidney stones, diarrhea, and a dependence on high doses. Acclimatization to high doses may cause symptoms of scurvy if the high doses are suddenly withdrawn.

**Vitamin C
(Ascorbic acid)**

FAT-SOLUBLE VITAMINS

The fat-soluble vitamins are **A, D, E,** and **K**. Unlike most of the water-soluble vitamins, where what isn't used gets excreted, any fat-soluble vitamins that are not used get stored. This means that excess A, D, E, and K can build up in your body to toxic levels. **For this reason taking excess fat-soluble vitamins is much more dangerous than taking excess water-soluble vitamins.**

However, it also means that many people are walking around with substantial storehouses of the fat-soluble vitamins (in their fat), and these folks are not in danger of becoming deficient in the fat-soluble vitamins anytime in the near future.

The fat-soluble vitamins require a small amount of dietary fat for absorption. People on Spartan "no-fat" diets run the risk of eventual fat-soluble vitamin deficiencies.

Vitamin A (Retinol)

Vitamin A, RDA: 1.0 mg (male), 0.8 mg (female)

Good sources: liver, eggs, cheese, butter, fortified margarine, milk, deep yellow vegetables (carrots, squash, cantaloupe), dark green vegetables (broccoli, spinach).

Vitamin A is important in the formation of skin, hair, and mucous membranes, for normal growth, and for night vision.

A deficiency of vitamin A causes rough skin, impaired growth, and night blindness or permanent blindness.

In one experiment, subjects were placed on a vitamin A-deficient diet for six months. Even on the deficient diets, blood vitamin A levels remained constant throughout the six-month period. No change was noted in physical performance. It is thought that liver stores of vitamin A may last for years in a well-fed person.

Excessive vitamin A may cause poor vision, nausea, vomiting, loss of appetite, peeling of skin, hair loss, fatigue, joint pain, bone abnormalities.

Vitamin D

Vitamin D, RDA: 0.075 mg (male), 0.075 mg (female)

Good sources: liver, cod liver oil, eggs, dairy products, fortified milk, margarine. Vitamin D is made in the skin upon contact with sunlight, but many people spend too little time in the sun or have skin too dark for this to be a significant source. The only foods that naturally contain vitamin D are oils. Milk often has vitamin D added to it.

Vitamin D is important for proper formation and mineralization of bones and teeth, and increases absorption of calcium.

In children, a deficiency of vitamin D causes **rickets**, a disease characterized by bone deformities, stunted growth, and poor teeth. In adults it causes **osteomalacia**, a disease characterized by progressive softening and bending of bones accompanied by shortened stature, frequent fractures, muscle spasms, and twitching.

Supplementation with excess vitamin D, either in moderate daily doses or in massive one-time doses, has not been shown to enhance physical performance.

Excessive vitamin D may cause calcium deposits throughout the body, deafness, nausea, vomiting, loss of appetite, high blood pressure, high blood cholesterol, kidney damage.

Vitamin E

Vitamin E, RDA: 10 mg (male), 8 mg (female)

Good sources: seeds, vegetable oils, margarines, whole-grain cereals and bread, liver, green leafy vegetables, peanuts, dairy products, wheat germ oil.

Vitamin E is important as an **antioxidant** (prevents other compounds from combining with oxygen), and so prevents cell membrane damage. It also is important in proper formation of red blood cells and muscles.

A deficiency of vitamin E is very difficult to produce, even in the laboratory, but based on animal studies it may cause reproductive failure, liver degeneration, heart damage, and muscular dystrophy.

Several well-controlled studies have shown that supplementation with vitamin E results in no improvement in aerobic or anaerobic performance under normal conditions. However, one study has shown improvements in aerobic performance at high altitudes (5,000 and 15,000 feet).

Excessive vitamin E, even though fat-soluble, has not clearly been shown to be a health hazard. However, there have been reports of headache, blurred vision, extreme fatigue, and muscle weakness.

Vitamin K

Vitamin K, RDA: 0.07-0.14 mg (male), 0.07-0.14 mg (female)

Good sources: green leafy vegetables, cabbage, cauliflower, liver, egg yolks, potatoes, and in small amounts in cereals, fruits, and meat. It is also produced by intestinal bacteria.

Vitamin K is important in blood clotting.

A deficiency of vitamin K can cause severe bleeding.

No studies concerning the effect of vitamin K on athletic performance have been done; however, there is no reason to think that a compound that facilitates blood clotting would have any particularly positive effects on physical performance.

Excessive vitamin K is relatively non-toxic, although synthetic forms may cause jaundice; in laboratory animals excessive vitamin K has produced anemia.

VITAMINS FOR PEAK PERFORMANCE

Some forty percent of the American population takes supplemental vitamins, including many athletes. Many of these athletes are taking them in search of the "competitive edge." They do this despite the fact that very few controlled studies have shown there to be any improvement in athletic performance from taking vitamins in excess of recommended amounts.

Why the persistent belief that vitamins enhance athletic performance, in the face of substantial evidence to the contrary? There *have* been some studies that have found improvements, but for the most part these studies are flawed. But these are often the only studies supplement manufacturers and distributors will cite.

Some valid studies have shown positive results in animal experiments or in humans in physiology labs; it is questionable to what degree these results are applicable to competing athletes. Furthermore, studies published in the last ten to fifteen years have generally failed to find differences between athletes given vitamins and those given placebos; these contrast with earlier, less well-controlled studies that did show differences. Experiments from Central and Eastern European countries showing positive results usually do not show positive results when repeated by American or British researchers.

Often, individuals who *did* show improvement with vitamin supplementation did so because they were deficient in vitamins to begin with. Since they were already below optimum vitamin levels, it is not surprising that for these people supplementation improved performance.

This does not mean that, for people who *are* at recommended vitamin levels, further vitamins would cause further improvements. It *does* mean that an athlete should ensure he or she gets adequate quantities of all vitamins. The recommended daily allowances are based on amounts of a vitamin necessary to prevent its specific deficiency disease, and are calculated by determining that amount, and adding a margin of safety. Although it can be argued that the amount required to prevent a deficiency disease is not necessarily the optimum amount for biological functioning, it has yet to be conclusively shown that amounts above the RDA promote better health than the RDA. (This may be in part because it is very difficult to measure "better health" in people who are already healthy.) This is an area of considerable controversy.

Because many athletes don't eat balanced diets, because moderate deficiencies can impair performance, and because vitamins are generally of low toxicity, multivitamin supplementation in amounts right around the RDA would seem a reasonable practice, if only as a form of "cheap insurance."

■ It is important to distinguish among having too little of a vitamin in your body (vitamin deficiency), having an appropriate amount of a vitamin in your body, and having too much of a vitamin in your body. If you give someone a vitamin they are deficient in, you may well see an improvement in athletic performance. This does not mean that vitamins will improve the performance of a person who is not deficient.

■ Because many athletes don't eat balanced diets, because moderate deficiencies can impair performance, and because vitamins are generally of low toxicity, multivitamin supplementation in amounts close to the RDA would seem a reasonable practice.

■ There is little conclusive evidence that vitamin doses above the RDA improve performance.

MINERALS

Minerals, like vitamins, are absolutely necessary for good health even though our bodies need them only in small amounts. Like vitamins, minerals have no calories. Unlike vitamins, minerals cannot be destroyed by cooking; however, they can be (and often are) *removed* from food during cooking or processing.

There are twenty-two minerals thought to be of biologic importance. Most are part of crucial enzyme systems, and participate in chemical reactions involving energy production, muscle movement, nerve function, and oxygen transport, to name a few.

Minerals fall into two groups: **major minerals** and **trace minerals**.

Major minerals are those needed in relatively large amounts, and include **calcium, phosphorus, sulfur, potassium, chloride, sodium,** and **magnesium.**

Trace minerals are those needed in tiny amounts, and include **iron, fluorine, zinc, copper, silicon, vanadium, tin, nickel, selenium, manganese, iodine, molybdenum, chromium, cobalt, lead,** and **arsenic.**

The functions and dietary requirements of the major minerals are much better understood than those of the trace minerals.

Minerals are present in all foods in varying amounts, but there may be geographical variations which change the mineral content of certain foods. For example, in some parts of the

United States (especially the Great Lakes Basin and the Pacific Northwest) the soil is poor in iodine. Because of this, certain vegetables grown in those regions have lower iodine content than the same vegetables grown elsewhere.

Like certain vitamins, minerals are toxic in excess doses. However, **the amount required for toxicity is much lower with minerals than with vitamins.** This makes megadosing (taking a nutrient in amounts exceeding ten times the RDA) with minerals particularly risky.

MAJOR MINERALS

Calcium

Calcium, RDA: 800 mg (male), 800 mg (female)

Good sources: Milk, cheese, dark green vegetables, peas, beans, sardines, canned salmon with bones. Calcium absorption from the intestines is impaired in diets high in phytates (a compound found in the bran of whole grains) and oxalates (a substance found in spinach, rhubarb, and beets).

Calcium is the most common mineral in the body, and is important for strong bones and teeth. It is also important for muscle contraction, proper nerve function, and blood clotting.

Calcium deficiency causes improper bone formation and stunted growth in children, and osteoporosis (weak, fracture-prone bones) in adults.

A diet high in protein (typical of many bodybuilders) increases losses of calcium in urine.

Excess calcium may cause drowsiness and lethargy, and interferes with absorption of iron, zinc, and manganese.

You need to maintain constant levels of calcium in your blood. If your blood calcium gets too low, there are homeostatic mechanisms for returning your calcium level to normal. These involve leeching calcium out of the bones so it can be used in the bloodstream, increasing intestinal absorption, and decreasing losses in the urine.

Similarly, if your blood calcium gets too high, there are homeostatic mechanisms for returning your calcium level to normal. This involves depositing more calcium in your bones and increasing the amount excreted in the urine.

There is currently much interest in the possibility of preventing or slowing osteoporosis in post-menopausal women by increasing the intake of dietary calcium. America's food processors have picked up on this quite quickly. Now you can buy all manner of calcium-fortified foods at your local supermarkets, such as calcium-fortified orange juice. At this point, the question of whether supplementation with calcium beyond the RDA does any good in the fight against osteoporosis has yet to be settled.

Strong bones, good nerve conduction, and good muscle contraction are all necessary for peak performance, so sufficient calcium from a variety of food sources should be part of every athlete's diet. There is no reason to think that excess calcium would have any positive effect on athletic performance.

Phosphorus

Phosphorus, RDA: 800 mg (male), 800 mg (female)

Good sources: Milk, cheese, meat, poultry, fish, dried beans and peas, soft drinks (as sodium phosphate), heavily processed foods

Phosphorus is the other major component of bone (along with calcium), so phosphorus is important for strong bones and teeth. In addition, phosphorus is the "P" in *ATP*, the *energy currency* of the body (see Chapter 13), so phosphorus participates in every energy-requiring step in the body. It also appears in DNA and RNA (genetic material), and cell membranes (as **phospholipids**).

Phosphorus deficiency can cause weakness and loss of calcium from bone.

As with calcium, you must maintain a constant level of phosphorus in your blood. If your blood phosphorus gets too high or too low, your kidneys homeostatically excrete more or less phosphorus as necessary to return blood phosphorus levels to normal.

Consuming excess phosphorus (easy to do for those who drink a lot of soft drinks) can cause a loss of calcium from bones. This may be a factor in the development of osteoporosis.

For athletes, dietary phosphorus deficiency is not a problem. In fact, *excess* phosphorus is more likely to be a problem. Athletes would be better off drinking fewer cans of soda and more glasses of fruit juice and milk.

Sulfur, RDA: none established

Good sources: high-protein foods—meat, eggs, dried beans and peas

Sulfur is necessary for the manufacture of connective tissue, the intercellular *glue* that holds other tissues together. It is also important for manufacture of cartilage and tendons, skin, hair, and nails.

Sulfur deficiency has not been observed in humans; excessive sulfur is thought to lead to poor growth.

Potassium, RDA: 1875-5100 mg (male), 1875-5100 mg (female)

Good sources: nuts, whole grains, meats, bananas, avocados, oranges, dried fruit, dried beans and peas

Potassium is one of the **electrolytes**, electrically-charged particles responsible for maintaining the right acid/base level and salt-and-water balance in the cells and fluid around the cells. (The other major electrolytes are sodium, chloride, and bicarbonate. Sodium and chloride are both minerals; we will discuss them in a moment.)

In addition to contributing to regulation of acid/base level and salt-and-water balance, potassium is also important for proper muscle contraction and nerve conduction.

Potassium deficiency can cause muscular weakness, paralysis, heart rhythm irregularities, lethargy, and kidney and lung failure.

Excess potassium can cause muscular weakness, paralysis, heart rhythm irregularities, and death.

Homeostatic mechanisms tightly control potassium levels, usually preventing the severe symptoms seen with potassium deficiency or excess. However, athletes who exercise for long periods in the heat, or who take diuretics, run the risk of potassium deficiency due to losses in sweat and urine. For these people, a potassium-containing sport drink, or a couple of extra bananas, may well be in order.

Chloride, RDA: 1700-5100 mg (male), 1700-5100 mg (female)

Good sources: table salt (sodium chloride), salt substitute (potassium chloride), processed foods

Sulfur

Potassium

Chloride

Like potassium, chloride is one of the **electrolytes**, electrically-charged particles responsible for maintaining the right acid/base level and salt-and-water balance in the cells and fluid around the cells.

Chloride is also a chief component of stomach acid, also called **hydro***chloric* acid.

Chloride deficiency, which is rare given the enormous quantity of salt most Americans eat, can cause muscle cramps, mental apathy, and reduced appetite.

Excessive chloride can cause vomiting and disturb the acid/base and salt-and-water balance.

Chloride is rarely talked about because it silently "tags along" with other minerals—it's the sodium in sodium chloride (table salt) that gets all the attention, and the potassium in potassium chloride (salt substitute) that gets talked about. Recently there has been some research suggesting that chloride itself, in addition to sodium, may play a role in high blood pressure.

Sodium

Sodium, RDA: 1100-3300 mg (male), 1100-3300 mg (female)

Good sources: table salt, processed foods

Like potassium and chloride, sodium is an *electrolyte*, an electrically-charged particle responsible for maintaining the right acid/base level and salt-and-water balance in the cells and fluid around the cells. Sodium is also important for proper nerve function.

Sodium deficiency can cause muscle cramps, mental apathy, and reduced appetite. However, sodium deficiency from insufficient sodium in the diet is not seen in the United States.

Excessive sodium causes high blood pressure in people who are susceptible; about twenty percent of Americans are susceptible. The average American consumes ten to twenty times more salt than necessary.

Athletes lose sodium in their sweat. However, sweating actually *increases* the concentration of sodium in the blood, because it causes you to lose more water than sodium (see Chapter 14). For this reason, *salt tablets are a bad idea*, unless taken under a doctor's supervision. Sweating increases blood sodium concentration above normal, and salt tablets only worsen the situation. Athletes don't need to be concerned about sodium loss in sweat until several hours into continuous hard exercise, and even then it is far more important to replenish lost water than lost sodium.

Magnesium

Magnesium, RDA: 350 mg (male), 300 mg (female)

Good sources: raw leafy green vegetables, whole grains, nuts, soybeans, seeds, cocoa

Sixty percent of the magnesium in your body is in your bones. Understandably, then, magnesium is important for strong, healthy bones. Magnesium also appears to stabilize energy release from food and muscle glycogen, facilitate transmission of nerve impulses to muscle, and assist in protein synthesis.

Magnesium deficiency can cause muscle cramps, weakness, spasms, irregular heart beat, growth impairment, and behavioral disturbances.

Excessive magnesium causes diarrhea and disturbed nervous system function.

TRACE MINERALS

Iron

Iron, RDA: 10 mg (male), 18 mg (female)

Good sources: meat, eggs, dried beans and peas, leafy green vegetables, whole grains, dried fruits

Iron is necessary in the formation of **hemoglobin**, the oxygen-carrying molecule in red blood cells, and **myoglobin**, a similar oxygen-carrying molecule in muscle. Iron also participates in several energy-releasing reactions.

When an untrained athlete begins training, the need for iron goes up. If there is not enough iron in the diet or in body iron stores, this increased need for iron may go unmet, resulting in suboptimum performance. Iron supplementation under these conditions improves performance.

Iron deficiency leads to impaired hemoglobin formation, which in turn leads to **anemia**, a condition of decreased oxygen-carrying capacity of the blood. Anemia is characterized by fatigue, weakness, pallor (unusually pale skin), and shortness of breath.

Anemia is very common among athletes, especially female athletes. Women are particularly at risk for iron deficiency anemia, because their iron requirements are greater, they get less iron in their diets, and they have significant menstrual iron losses.

Long-distance runners are also at risk. For reasons that are not fully understood, long-distance runners often bleed from the stomach and intestines. This is exacerbated by stomach-irritating medications such as aspirin, ibuprofen (Advil), and indomethacin (Indocin), medications that runners often take for minor injuries and inflammation. In one study of joggers and competition runners, over half the subjects were iron deficient, and one-fifth had iron deficiency anemia, in part from blood losses from the stomach and intestines. **After supplementation, virtually all deficiencies were corrected, and performance times improved.**

Stomach and intestinal bleeding often have no symptoms at all, so long-distance runners can get an iron-deficiency anemia unknowingly.

It is important to distinguish between **iron deficiency anemia** and **sports anemia**. **Iron deficiency anemia** is a decrease in blood oxygen-carrying capacity caused by insufficient iron in the diet or by blood loss. **Sports anemia** is a decrease in blood oxygen-carrying capacity associated with heavy physical exertion. For whatever reason, people who engage in heavy physical exertion decrease their oxygen-carrying capacity. Since sports anemia is not caused by insufficient iron, it is not surprising that iron supplementation does not remedy sports anemia.

Athletes may lose significant amounts of iron in sweat, especially in hot climates, and may consequently need more iron in their diets than non-athletes.

Although iron supplementation clearly improves the performances of athletes with suboptimal iron intakes, it appears to be of little good to athletes who have normal iron intakes.

Excessive iron intake leads to deposition of iron in the liver, pancreas, and heart, which can impair the function of all of these organs.

Zinc

Zinc, RDA: 15 mg (male), 15 mg (female)

Good sources: beef, liver, dark turkey and dark chicken meat, oysters. Zinc is present in many vegetable sources as well, such as whole grains and cereals, nuts, and peanuts, but these sources also contain phytate and certain dietary fibers that may interfere with absorption of zinc from the intestines.

Zinc plays an important role in more than one hundred enzymes, helping to maintain normal protein, fat, and carbohydrate metabolism.

Zinc deficiency causes decreased taste sensation, loss of appetite, delayed wound healing, impaired cell growth, and impaired immune defenses. By some estimates much of the U.S. population is getting one-half the RDA or less.

Excessive zinc intake causes nausea, vomiting, anemia, bleeding from the stomach, abdominal pain, and fever.

Exercise increases zinc losses in urine, and losses in sweat can be significant as well. Supplementation should be done carefully, if at all, as symptoms of toxicity appear at levels not much above the RDA.

Copper, RDA: 2-3 mg (male), 2-3 mg (female)

Good sources: shellfish, nuts, liver, kidneys, dried beans, potatoes. High intakes of simple sugars (including honey) impair copper metabolism

Copper plays a key role in a number of processes in the body, including energy production, fat metabolism, red blood cell formation, and connective tissue formation.

Prolonged marginal copper intake can cause anemia, loss of tendon and artery elasticity, and bone demineralization. The typical American diet contains only about half the RDA.

Exercise increases copper losses in stool, sweat, and urine. Sweat losses can be considerable: in hot, humid environments, almost half of the daily copper intake can be lost in sweat.

Exercise increases blood levels of copper, a change that persists even at rest. This increase is thought to be due to increased levels of copper-containing proteins including **cytochrome oxidase**, the enzyme responsible for one of the last steps in the energy production process.

Increased copper losses, coupled with inadequate intake, may result in marginal serum copper levels, This may alter the pathways of fat metabolism and energy production, possibly affecting performance. However, no cause-and-effect relationship between marginal serum copper levels and athletic performance has yet been demonstrated.

As with zinc, supplementation should be done carefully, if at all, as copper is toxic at levels not much above the RDA.

Copper

Chromium

Chromium, RDA: 0.050-0.200 mg (male), 0.050-0.200 mg (female)

Good sources: mushrooms, oysters, black pepper, brewer's yeast, apples with skins, wine, beer

The physiologic role of chromium has yet to be fully elucidated; however, chromium clearly has a role in the regulation of carbohydrate and lipid (fat) metabolism, primarily by affecting the action of insulin.

Chromium deficiency may cause abnormal carbohydrate and lipid metabolism, impaired glucose tolerance, elevated serum insulin, and elevated cholesterol and triglycerides. Up to ninety percent of Americans may be getting less than the RDA. In addition, diets high in simple sugars, as are most American diets, can increase losses of chromium in the urine by as much as 300%.

Exercise also increases chromium losses. Intense exercise can increase losses of chromium in the urine fivefold; however, athletes appear to compensate for these losses to some degree. Trained runners excrete significantly less chromium on non-exercise days than do inactive people, suggesting an athletic adaptation that increases the ability to conserve chromium.

Chromium has been shown to cause skin and kidney damage from occupational exposure, but the effects of dietary excess are not known. There is no evidence that megadosing with chromium provides any health or athletic benefits.

Fluorine

Fluorine, RDA: 1.5-4.0 mg (male), 1.5-4.0 mg (female)

Good sources: drinking water (especially fluoridated drinking water), tea, seafood, anything prepared with fluorinated water

Fluorine is important in the formation of strong bones and teeth, and decreases the incidence of cavities.

Fluorine deficiency leads to increased cavities, and may contribute to osteoporosis, poor growth, and anemia.

Excessive fluorine intake causes mottling of teeth, increased bone density, and disturbances of the nervous system. In large doses, fluorine is poisonous.

There is little known about the role of fluorine in athletic performance.

Silicon, RDA: not established

Good sources: high-fiber foods, drinking water

Silicon has only recently (1972) been recognized as a necessary nutrient. Not much is known about it, but it appears to be important in the formation of skin, cartilage, elastic tissue, and collagen.

A comparison of two populations of Finns showed those with twice the silicon in their drinking water had half the long-term rate of heart disease. Other researchers have found that the more the silicon content of an artery wall, the less hardening of the arteries is present. Thus silicon appears to provide some kind of protection against heart disease, and silicon deficiency may be a contributing factor in hardening of the arteries.

Since silicon is found in high-fiber foods, and fiber intake is associated with decreased heart disease, it may be that fiber decreases heart disease by providing a source of silicon in the diet.

Occupational exposure of silicon causes silicosis, a lung disease caused by chronic inhalation of silicon-containing stone and cement dust, but there is no evidence for a dietary silicon toxicity.

There is no known association between silicon and athletic performance.

Vanadium, RDA: unknown

Good sources: vanadium content of various foods is not known

Vanadium is another recent (1971) addition to the nutritional arsenal, and falls into the category of *probably essential*. Vanadium appears to play a role in the regulation of fat metabolism, ATP metabolism, and bone mineralization. Animal experiments have shown vanadium to suppress cholesterol synthesis, thus lowering cholesterol levels; this has not been borne out with experiments in humans.

Since so little is known, it is unclear which foods are good sources, how much gets absorbed, how much is needed, or how much constitutes an excess. Nothing is known of vanadium and athletic performance.

Silicon

Vanadium

Tin

Tin, RDA: unknown

Good sources: food packaged in tin cans

Another newcomer (1970), tin has been shown to produce dramatic growth increases in rats who previously had been on "tin-free" diets. How it produces these effects is unknown.

It is unclear what symptoms, if any, there are of tin deficiency.

Tin toxicity from excess intake is quite rare, as tin is poorly absorbed from the intestines.

There is no information available on tin and athletic performance.

Nickel

Nickel, RDA: unknown

Good sources: plants

Nickel probably plays a role in energy production in the **mitochondria** (the *powerhouse of the cell*).

Nickel deficiency changes the structure of liver cells and mitochondria, and results in decreased levels of several mitochondrial enzymes necessary for energy production. Nickel deficiency also decreases iron absorption.

In animal studies, chronic excess nickel intake has been shown to cause degeneration of heart muscle, brain, lung, liver, and kidney.

There is no information available on nickel and athletic performance.

Selenium

Selenium, RDA: 0.05-0.2 mg (male), 0.05-0.2 mg (female)

Good sources: Seafood, meat, grains, garlic, mushrooms, asparagus

Selenium has attracted quite a bit of attention recently, as diets low in selenium have been linked with higher rates of cancer of the colon, rectum, prostate, breast, tongue, esophagus, stomach, intestine, liver, pancreas, bladder, and lung.

Selenium is important in the manufacture of the antioxidant **glutathione**. Like its fellow antioxidants vitamin C and vitamin E, glutathione functions to protect cell membranes from the toxic effects of exercise.

Selenium deficiency may cause anemia in man; in animals it has been shown to cause growth retardation and cataract formation. Dietary deficiencies are rare.

There is no information available on selenium and athletic performance.

Manganese, RDA: not established

Good sources: nuts, whole grains, green leafy vegetables, fruits, tea, instant coffee, cocoa powder

Manganese is an essential component of many enzymes, including enzymes involved with energy production and fat synthesis.

Manganese deficiency interferes with normal nervous system function, reproduction, and growth and maintenance of connective tissue, cartilage, and bone.

High doses can cause neurologic abnormalities.

Manganese

Iodine, RDA: 0.15 mg (males), 0.15 mg (females)

Good sources: marine fish, shellfish, iodized salt, sea salt, seaweed, meat, eggs, dairy products. Iodine content of food varies considerably depending on iodine content of soil and fertilizer and degree of processing the food undergoes.

Iodine is a necessary component of the thyroid hormones, which serve to regulate your metabolic rate and oxygen consumption, and appear to play a role in protein synthesis and release of fat from fat stores.

Iodine deficiency causes a decline of circulating thyroid hormone levels, and reduces metabolic rate. Severe iodine deficiency causes **goiter**, an enlargement of the thyroid gland in the neck.

The average American consumes about five times the RDA of iodine. Moderately high iodine intake (ten to twenty times the RDA) is not known to cause any health problems, although very high intake may depress activity of the thyroid gland.

An iodine deficiency can interfere with athletic performance by lowering metabolic rate. This can be corrected with supplementation, but iodine in excess of the RDA does not further enhance performance. Since the average American intake is about five times the RDA, for most people supplementation seems unnecessary.

Iodine

Molybdenum

Molybdenum, RDA: not established

Good sources: dried beans and peas, peanuts, lentils, cereal grains, liver, kidneys

Molybdenum is an important constituent of several enzymes, including enzymes in the protein breakdown chain.

Molybdenum deficiency is not known in humans, but in animals it has been shown to cause growth retardation and death.

Dietary molybdenum interferes with intestinal absorption of copper and iron. In rare instances, excess molybdenum intake may cause a copper deficiency.

There is no information available on molybdenum and athletic performance.

Cobalt

Cobalt, RDA: required as vitamin B12

Good sources: vegetables, whole grains

Cobalt is found in vitamin B12, and is necessary for vitamin B12 to function properly. It is unclear whether cobalt serves any essential functions outside of its role in B12.

Cobalt deficiency has never been documented, even in animals.

Excess cobalt may have a toxic effect on the heart, and there have been several reported cases of death associated with excess cobalt intake. (Cobalt used to be added to a particular brand of beer to enhance foaming; these deaths were seen in people who drank a lot of that beer.)

There is no information available on cobalt and athletic performance.

Lead

Lead, RDA: not established

Good sources: widely distributed in foods, especially those grown near highways. Content in canned foods is relatively high, especially evaporated milk, where lead solder is still used. Lead is one of the few trace minerals that is not removed in refining of wheat products. Calcium supplements made with bone meal may be quite high in lead.

Lead has quite recently (1979) been found to be necessary for good health. It is necessary in very tiny amounts, however, and it is still poisonous in large amounts.

Interestingly, lead has both its beneficial and poisonous effects on blood. A lead deficiency produces anemia, reduces iron absorption, and reduces iron stores in liver and spleen. Excess lead also causes anemia, but also causes kidney damage, hyperactivity and other behavioral problems in children, and impaired intellectual development.

The average American intake is probably far in excess of what is needed. Avoiding a toxic level is the important concern; deficiency is not a problem. Lead intake is probably declining, as less and less leaded gasoline is sold, and as increased use of glass jars and seamless aluminum cans (with decreased use of leaded cans) is seen.

Arsenic, RDA: not established

Good sources: seafood, especially shellfish and shrimp, some drinking water

Arsenic has been shown to be necessary for good health in laboratory animals, but it is still unclear if it is necessary for good health in humans. In animals, arsenic deficiency causes red blood cells to become fragile, break apart, and die early, and causes anemia and impaired growth.

The role of arsenic in normal functioning is not known, but it is concentrated in the proteins of skin, hair, and fingernails, and may play a role in normal formation of these tissues. It also interacts with certain proteins and enzymes.

Although one researcher has suggested that the average American intake may be inadequate, others feel arsenic poisoning still remains a greater threat than arsenic deficiency. Selenium excess has been shown to deplete body arsenic, and vice versa.

Excess arsenic intake is characterized by weakness, muscle aches, nerve abnormalities, decreased thyroid function.

Arsenic

The role of trace minerals is probably the least-understood area in nutrition today.

A variety of minerals are being recognized as necessary for good health, including some, such as lead and arsenic, which not long ago were dismissed as uniformly poisonous. It is likely that in the future more minerals will come to be recognized as necessary for good health. This is one of many reasons

CONCLUSIONS

a balanced diet is so important. It does not make sound nutritional sense to eat a poor diet while taking every supplement known to man, blithely assuming the supplements are adequately compensating for other nutritional indiscretions.

Only with a balanced diet, eating a variety of foods, can you reasonably ensure adequate nutrition.

This is not to say all supplements are bad. While repeated studies have shown that taking minerals in excess of the RDA does not improve athletic performance, many mineral deficiencies impair athletic performance. Given that, even with a good diet, some minerals are difficult to get in amounts recommended for good health, it is reasonable to take a multivitamin/multimineral supplement that supplies amounts close to the RDA. **Megadosing** is dangerous, however, especially with minerals, and is not recommended.

■ **Minerals are essential for good health, even though our bodies need them only in small amounts.**

■ **Minerals can be categorized into two groups: *major minerals* and *trace minerals*.**

❏ **Major minerals are those needed in relatively large amounts, and include calcium, phosphorus, sulfur, potassium, chloride, sodium, and magnesium.**

❏ **Trace minerals are those needed in tiny amounts, and include iron, fluorine, zinc, copper, silicon, vanadium, tin, nickel, selenium, manganese, iodine, molybdenum, chromium, cobalt, lead, and arsenic.**

■ Minerals are toxic in excess doses.

  ❑ Toxicity levels are much lower with minerals than with vitamins.

■ Deficiencies of certain minerals will prevent optimum athletic performance.

■ Excess intake of many minerals (amounts above and beyond the RDA's) has been shown to have *no positive effect on athletic performance.*

■ Guidelines for Optimum Sports Nutrition:

  ❑ Since regional soil variations may make it difficult to get even the RDA's of some minerals from a balanced diet, and since mineral deficiencies do impair athletic performance, we recommend taking a multimineral tablet with dosages close to the RDA's.

  ❑ Given the high risk of toxicity for many minerals, and the evidence of lack of improvement in athletic performance from mineral intake in excess of the RDA's, we strongly recommend against taking megadoses of minerals.

❖   ❖   ❖

SPECIAL NUTRITIONAL TOPICS

So far, we've looked at the major categories of nutrients and at what happens to those nutrients in the body. This chapter examines other substances of special concern: **fiber, cholesterol, salt**, and **sugar**. Understanding each of these subjects is important both for your general health and your ability to perform.

FIBER

Only in recent years has fiber become a major nutritional topic. In the early 1970's, researchers advanced the "dietary fiber hypothesis," which theorized a connection between low fiber intake and a high incidence of certain diseases—including colon cancer, coronary heart disease, diabetes, and hypertension.

While the studies underlying this theory demonstrated only statistical correlations—not cause and effect—continuing research seems to support the dietary fiber hypothesis with regard to certain diseases.

What Is Fiber?

Dietary fiber refers to a family of carbohydrate substances which are not broken down by intestinal enzymes. Because they are not broken down, they pass intact into the colon. Fiber only comes from plant sources, and is the indigestible remnants of plant cells.

Fiber is usually divided into two categories: **water insoluble** ("scratchy") and **water soluble** ("gummy"). Wheat, vegetables, and most grain fibers contain mostly insoluble fibers, such as cellulose and lignin. Fruits, oats, and legumes contain mostly soluble fibers, such as pectin, gums, and mucilages.

What Does Fiber Do?

Both soluble fiber and insoluble fiber absorb many times their weight in water. This increases the "bulk" of the material that is passing through the intestines, resulting in more-frequent bowel movements, softer stools, and faster passage through the intestines. Thus both kinds of fiber are natural laxatives.

Both kinds also delay glucose absorption from the small intestine. This tends to "smoothe out" the delivery of glucose to the blood, so the bloodstream doesn't get hit with a huge dose of sugar all at once.

Dietary fiber alters the bacterial metabolism that takes place in your colon. It may bind or dilute cancer-causing agents, and may alter the metabolism of bile acid. It is these and other potential effects, still under intense study, that suggest fiber may lower the risk of colon cancer.

Not all of the fiber you eat passes out in the stools. Although the fiber passes undigested from the small intestine into the colon, about eighty percent of the fiber in your diet gets broken down in your colon by the bacteria that reside there.

What Are The Benefits of Eating Fiber?

For Diabetics

High fiber diets can be very good for persons with diabetes. Research has shown that such diets improve the diabetics' blood sugar control, lower their insulin requirements, and decrease their serum cholesterol concentrations compared to more typical diets.

For People with High Cholesterol Levels

Similar good results have been obtained for people with unacceptably high blood cholesterol or triglyceride (fat) levels. For them, a diet high in soluble fiber—achieved primarily by adding oat bran and beans—lowers the LDL level, raises the HDL level, and lowers serum triglycerides in both the short and long term. (More on LDL's and HDL's later on in this chapter.)

Fiber and Heart Disease

Scientists also believe high fiber intake reduces your risk of coronary heart disease. Just how it does this is unclear—it seems to be something other than just the positive effect on serum cholesterol, perhaps having to do with the trace mineral *silicon* in fiber—but the statistics are hard to ignore: Japan, with the highest fiber intake among the developed countries, has the lowest rate of coronary heart disease. The United States, with the lowest intake of dietary fiber, has the highest rate of coronary heart disease. These figures don't prove cause and effect, but are highly suggestive.

Fiber and Weight Loss

Fiber also appears to promote weight loss, for several reasons.

First, fiber slows the movement of food from the stomach to the small intestine, enhancing the feeling of fullness, and making it easier to limit the intake of food.

Second, it physically takes longer to eat fibrous food (such as apples) than non-fibrous food (such as apple juice), so less gets eaten.

Third, it may take more energy to absorb and digest high-fiber foods than it does low-fiber foods.

Researchers are still investigating the proper role of fiber in overall health. Not all the results are in. However, in addition to the areas already discussed, a number of other *potential* benefits from fiber are the subjects of current research. Fiber:

- may help maintain lower blood pressure
- may reduce the incidence of a number of gastrointestinal problems, such as gallstones, appendicitis, constipation, and hemorrhoids
- may reduce the incidence of colon cancer

Fiber can have a down side, though. It may decrease the availability of certain nutrients—the minerals calcium, zinc, iron, magnesium, phosphorus, copper, and possibly vitamin B12. Fiber also increases the production of intestinal gas in some people, but this effect disappears after a few weeks.

The Down Side

The average American diet contains about ten grams of fiber. The National Cancer Institute recommends increasing that to twenty to thirty grams.

Where should you get all this fiber? Start with breakfast cereal. High fiber cereals are a growing segment of the cereal market, and many are excellent sources of fiber. But read the box before you buy. The amount of fiber per serving varies significantly among the various cereals (see Table on next page), and many cereals are quite high in sugar.

Because both water-soluble and water-insoluble fiber have unique benefits, your daily diet should include sources of both. You should get ample quantities if you include fresh fruits and vegetables, beans, whole-grain breads, and nuts and seeds in your diet. The following chart shows some good sources of fiber.

How Much Is Enough?

SELECTED SOURCES OF DIETARY FIBER

FOOD AND AMOUNT	GRAMS OF FIBER (approx.)
Pork and Beans (1/2 cup)	11.0
Dry-roasted Unsalted Peanuts (1/2 cup)	10.0
Garbanzo Beans (1/2 cup)	8.0
Kidney Beans (1/2 cup)	8.0
Brazil Nuts (1/2 cup)	5.4
Raisins (1/2 cup)	5.2
Raspberries (1/2 cup)	4.6
Dried Fig (1)	3.7
Guava (1)	3.6
Sweet Potato (1)	3.5
Barley (1/2 cup, cooked)	3.0
Papaya (1)	2.8
Eggplant (1/2 cup)	2.5
Prune (1)	2.0
Watermelon (1 cup)	1.4
Dried Apricot (1)	1.0

FIBER CONTENT OF SELECTED CEREALS

CEREAL	GRAMS FIBER PER 1 OZ. SERVING
Kellog's All-bran with Extra Fiber	13.0
General Mills Fiber One	12.0
Nabisco 100% Bran	10.0
Kellog's All-Bran	9.0
Kellog's Bran Buds	8.0
Post Natural Bran Flakes	5.0
Quaker Corn Bran	5.0
Kellog's Crackling O's	4.0
Shredded Wheat	3.0
Raisin Bran	2.0

■ *Fiber* refers to the indigestible remnants of plant cells.

■ There are two kinds of fiber: water-soluble and water- insoluble.

❏ An increased intake of *insoluble* fiber appears to lower the risk of colon cancer.

❏ An increased intake of *soluble* fiber appears to lower the risk of coronary heart disease and high serum cholesterol.

❏ Both soluble and insoluble fiber enhance the sense of "fullness," and both are useful for losing weight.

■ Good sources include: Cereals, fruits, vegetables, beans, whole-grain breads, nuts and seeds.

CHOLESTEROL

What is Cholesterol?

Cholesterol is a widely misunderstood substance. Indeed, many people don't realize that the body *needs* cholesterol to function properly. Let's take a look at cholesterol's biochemical role, and how issues related to cholesterol figure into a nutritional program.

Cholesterol is a **steroid**. In fact, it's the most abundant steroid in the body.* Cholesterol is found in the membrane of every cell in your body. Cholesterol is *not* found in any plant cell membranes. So fruit and vegetables contain no cholesterol at all.

What Does Cholesterol Do?

Cholesterol is necessary for normal functioning in a number of ways:

■ As a component of all animal cell membranes, it helps the membranes maintain the appropriate degree of "fluidity" they need to operate properly.

■ It is the substance from which your body produces vitally important hormones, such as cortisone, aldosterone, and vitamin D.

■ It is used in large amounts by your liver in producing **bile salts**, which are central to fat absorption in the small intestine.

Why Be Concerned About Cholesterol?

High levels of cholesterol in the blood are strongly associated with increased rates of atherosclerotic heart disease (hardening of the arteries, a condition which contributes to more than half of all deaths in the United States). Diets high in cholesterol have also been linked with increased rates of atherosclerotic heart disease, but there is controversy surrounding how closely cholesterol in the *diet* is related to cholesterol in the *blood*. Most of the cholesterol in the blood is manufactured by the liver, and it is unclear to what extent the total blood cholesterol can be affected by diet.

---

*This is steroid in the true biochemical usage, not in the limited athletic sense. See Chapter 13 for more on steroids.

Lipoproteins

Much of the recent focus on cholesterol has centered on the **lipoproteins**, especially **LDL's** and **HDL's**. Lipoproteins are transport vehicles for fat and cholesterol. Since oil and water don't mix, fat and cholesterol can't be transported in a controlled manner if they are simply floating free in the water-based blood. They need a vehicle for transport, and lipoproteins are that vehicle.

Lipoproteins are so-called because they contain both lipids (fats) and protein. They are assembled in your intestinal tract and liver, then sent out to circulate through your bloodstream.

A Question of Density

Lipoproteins are classified into four groups: **chylomicrons**, **VLDL's, LDL's**, and **HDL's**.

Chylomicrons. Chylomicrons contain about ninety percent dietary triglycerides and about five percent cholesterol, and are responsible for carrying the fat you eat to fat cells and the cholesterol you eat to the liver. The number of chylomicrons in the blood goes up temporarily after a fatty meal.

VLDL's. VLDL's (for *very low density lipoproteins*) contain about sixty percent triglycerides and twelve percent cholesterol. VLDL's are responsible for carrying fats manufactured in the liver (*not* dietary fats) to fat cells.

LDL's. Once the VLDL releases its fat molecules into a fat cell, the lipoprotein particle contains proportionately more cholesterol and less fat; this particle is now called an LDL (for *low density lipoprotein*).

LDL's contain about ten percent triglycerides and about fifty percent cholesterol; about three-quarters of all the cholesterol in your bloodstream is contained in LDL's. LDL's are responsible for supplying cholesterol to cells in your body that need them.

HDL's. The fourth group is the HDL's (for *high density lipoproteins*). These contain mostly **phospholipids**—lipids containing phosphorus—and are only about twenty percent cholesterol and five percent triglycerides. HDL's are responsible for removing cholesterol from cells and the bloodstream and returning it to the liver and LDL's.

"Good" and "Bad" Lipoproteins

In general terms, VLDL's and especially LDL's are the "bad" lipoproteins, while HDL's are the "good" lipopoteins. A high level of LDL's has been associated with increased rates of atherosclerotic heart disease, especially in the presence of high blood pressure, smoking, diabetes, or obesity. A high level of HDL's has been associated with decreased rates of atherosclerotic heart disease. **The upshot of all this is that you want to lower the level of LDL's in your blood and raise the level of HDL's.**

The first thing you can do is *exercise*. For reasons not yet understood, exercise—especially intense aerobic exercise—raises HDL levels.

The second thing you can do is alter your diet.

As mentioned above, there is controversy surrounding how closely cholesterol in the diet is related to cholesterol in the blood. Many studies have demonstrated strong associations between cholesterol intake and death from atherosclerotic heart disease. On the other hand, some people can eat large quantities of cholesterol without experiencing concomitant increases in blood cholesterol levels or atherosclerotic heart disease. It's likely that not all people are equally sensitive to the amount of cholesterol in their diet; in other words, the same amount of cholesterol in the diet may raise the blood cholesterol level of one person and not another. More research needs to be done to clarify this.

How Can I Improve My Cholesterol Levels?

Dietary Cholesterol

CHOLESTEROL CONTENT OF SELECTED FOODS

FOOD AND AMOUNT	MG. CHOLESTEROL (approx.)
Liver (3.5 ounce serving)	300
Lobster (3.5 ounce serving)	200
Egg (1)	274
Cheddar Cheese (3.5 ounces)	105
Chicken (3.5 ounce serving)	88
Ice Cream (1 cup)	80
Beef (3.5 ounce serving)	70
Lamb (3.5 ounce serving)	70
Fish (3.5 ounce serving)	60
Ham (3.5 ounce serving)	58
Whole Milk (1 cup)	35
Butter (1 tsp.)	11

Meanwhile, until a more definitive answer is available, it is reasonable to lower the intake of cholesterol-rich foods in your diet and monitor the cholesterol levels in your blood. The American Heart Association recommends reducing dietary cholesterol intake to below 300 milligrams/day (the current intake is 450 mg/day).

The table on the previous page will help you assess your intake of dietary cholesterol.

Dietary Fat

Only ten percent of the cholesterol in your blood comes directly from diet; the other ninety percent is manufactured by your liver. Even more significant than dietary cholesterol in determining your blood cholesterol is the amount of **fat** in your diet. This fact is the basis for several nutritional recommendations:

■ First, recall from Chapter 6 that only twenty to thirty percent of your total calories should come from fat. Most people consume much more than that, and in so doing elevate their LDL levels. So keeping your over-

SOME COMMON SOURCES OF DIETARY FAT

FOOD AND AMOUNT	GRAMS OF FAT (approx.)
Meat and Fish	
Pork Sausage (3 ounces)	36
Beef, Pork, or Lamb, cooked with fat trimmed (3 ounces)	20
Fish (3 ounces, broiled)	6
Chicken (3 ounces, roasted without skin)	4
Dairy Products	
Ice Cream (1 cup)	30
Swiss or Cheddar Cheese (1 ounce)	9
Whole Milk (1 cup)	8
Egg (1)	6
Lowfat Milk (2%) (1 cup)	5
Butter (1 tsp.)	4
Low-fat Yogurt (1 cup)	3
Skim Milk (1 cup)	.4

all fat intake down is the first important step. The table on the previous page shows some of the more common sources of dietary fat.

■ Second, recall also that a maximum of ten percent of your total calories (one half or less of your total fat intake) should come from *saturated* fats. The remainder should come from *monounsaturated* and *polyunsaturated* fats.

The reason is simple: saturated fats *raise* the level of LDL's, while mono- and polyunsaturated fats tend to *lower* the level of LDL's. Furthermore, there is mounting evidence that monounsaturated fats, unlike polyunsaturated ones, may lower LDL's without also lowering HDL's.

So, use as little fats and oils as possible. When you do use oils, it may be advisable to use monounsaturated oils such as olive oil, avocado oil, and peanut oil. The table below can help you make the best choices.

APPROXIMATE FATTY ACID CONTENT OF SELECTED VEGETABLE OILS

TYPE OF OIL	% SATURATED	% POLYUNSATURATED	% MONOUNSATURATED
Canola Oil	6	32	62
Corn Oil	15	59	26
Olive Oil	14	9	77
Peanut Oil	18	34	48
Safflower Oil	9	75	16
Sesame Oil	20	40	40
Sunflower Oil	11	22	67

■ Third, watch out for *hidden* fats and oils. Some foods you may not think of as fatty—such as avocados and coconuts—actually contain lots of fat. Other foods—such as non-dairy creamers and packaged cookies—are processed with highly saturated coconut and palm oils.

■ Finally, watch for labels stating that a product includes *partially hydrogenated* oils. Remember, hydrogenation is a process that makes oils more saturated.

That's better for shelf life, but not for your health, as saturated oils raise blood cholesterol levels. The table below identifies some of the sources of hidden fats.

SOME "HIDDEN" SOURCES OF DIETARY FAT

FOOD AND AMOUNT	GRAMS OF FAT (approx.)
Pecans (1/2 cup)	42
Avocado (1)	37
Peanuts (1/2 cup)	36
Vegetable Oil (1 tablespoon)	14
Tuna Salad (1/2 cup)	10.5
Bran Muffin (1 small)	5.1
Mayonnaise (1 tsp.)	3.7
Doughnut (1)	6

Fish Oil

Fish oil is another nutritional item getting a lot of attention these days. Although it appears to offer a number of potential benefits, keep in mind that the research is still in a very early stage, and scientists are not ready to make unequivocal statements about it yet.

Omega-3 Fatty Acids

The whole fish oil craze can be traced to the Eskimos. In the early 1970's, some Danish researchers noticed that the Greenland Eskimos, who ate almost no carbohydrates but consumed large amounts of fat, suffered virtually no coronary artery disease. This started the scientists thinking, and led to the discovery that many cold-water fish contain **omega-3 fatty acids**.

Omega-3 fatty acids appear to have two major effects on the body, each of which may lower the risk of death from heart disease:

- They seem to be even more effective than other unsaturated fats at reducing LDL and triglyceride levels in normal individuals. (As we saw above, lower LDL and triglyceride levels are associated with a lower incidence of heart disease.)

  Their effect on HDL levels varies.

■ They appear to induce changes in platelet function and vascular reactivity—meaning that they increase bleeding time, but decrease platelet adhesiveness and platelet count. Although these changes do not directly change the course of heart disease, they do lessen the chance of getting a blood clot in a coronary artery, and so lessen the chance of a heart attack.

Does fish oil have a down side? In theory it might, but in practice it need not.

The Down Side

Increasing polyunsaturated fat intake increases the need for Vitamin E; so, in theory, you could develop a Vitamin E deficiency by consuming large amounts of fish oil. However, a properly balanced diet, including grains and leafy green vegetables, supplies enough Vitamin E to offset this possibility.

It's also theoretically possible that a high fish oil diet might dangerously prolong bleeding time. This problem has not been reported, however, and does not appear to be cause for concern.

Dosage. Although experts disagree on the optimum daily intake, the current recommendation is four to eight grams per day. That amount seems to provide the maximum benefit, without unnecessarily raising overall fat intake.

How Much Fish Oil Do I Need, And What Are The Best Sources?

Even smaller amounts, however, should result in some amount of benefit. The omega-3 fatty acids are present in many fish—salmon and mackerel being the most generous sources—

SELECTED SOURCES OF OMEGA-3 FATTY ACIDS

SOURCE	GR. OMEGA-3 F.A. PER 100 GR. SOURCE
MaxEPA Oil	29.4
Salmon Oil	20.9
Cod Liver Oil	19.2
Walnut Oil	10.4
Dried Butternuts	8.7
Soybean Oil	6.8
Atlantic Mackerel	2.6
Butter	1.2

and are also found in some non-fish foods. See the table on the previous page for a listing of sources.

Fish Oil Supplements vs. Dietary Sources. Next question is whether taking fish oil supplements is a good way to get omega-3 fatty acids. The answer: no one knows. The studies showing beneficial changes in cholesterol and triglyceride levels have all been done using dietary fish oils from fish, *not* fish oil capsules.

Most fish oil capsules don't have much fish oil in them, and so you are probably better off just eating fish a few times a week. (But don't deep-fry it! You'll defeat the purpose of eating the omega-3 fish oils if you overload on other fats at the same time.)

- Cholesterol performs vital functions in the body.

- Cholesterol is manufactured in the liver and supplied by the diet. Enough is made in the liver that you don't need any in the diet.

- Elevated blood cholesterol, elevated low-density lipoproteins (LDL's), and decreased high-density lipoproteins (HDL's) are associated with increased risk of heart disease.

- Cutting down on cholesterol consumption appears to decrease the risk of heart disease. The recommendation from the National Cancer Institute calls for decreasing cholesterol consumption by one-third (from 450 milligrams cholesterol per day to 300mg./day).

- It is also possible to reduce blood cholesterol by reducing overall fat intake, reducing saturated fat intake, and eating proportionately more mono- and polyunsaturated fats.

- Eating more of certain kinds of fish, in order to consume more omega-3 fatty acids, may also lower cholesterol level.

SALT

Salt is another misunderstood substance that gets a lot of attention among the nutrition-conscious. Like cholesterol, salt is necessary for proper body functioning. And as with cholesterol, problems can arise from consuming too much of it.

What is Salt?

Ordinary table salt is **sodium chloride**. For nutritional purposes, when we talk about salt, we're really talking about the *sodium* part of sodium chloride. (Technically, potassium chloride is also a salt, but since it is really the sodium that we are concerned with, the term *salt* as used here will refer only to sodium chloride.)

What Does Salt (OK, *Sodium*) Do?

Sodium accounts for only two percent of the minerals in your body, but nonetheless is widely distributed: it is in the fluid that surrounds every cell in your body. It teams with potassium to facilitate the flow of nutrients into your cells, and of waste back out again.

Sodium performs a number of other vital functions. It:

- helps maintain the pH balance (relative acidity or alkalinity) of your blood and other bodily tissues
- is part of the system that helps the transfer of glucose through your intestinal walls into your blood stream
- is necessary for proper nerve conduction
- helps maintain proper fluid pressure in your cells
- helps your stomach make hydrochloric acid

What Happens if I Eat Too Much Salt?

You need a certain concentration of sodium in your blood at all times. This concentration is maintained within fairly narrow homeostatic boundaries by your kidneys.

If the concentration falls below the lower boundary, a substance called ACTH (**adrenocorticotropic hormone**, produced by your pituitary gland) stimulates your adrenal glands to produce another hormone called **aldosterone**. Aldosterone tells your kidneys to retrieve sodium from urine and return it to your blood.

On the other hand, if the concentration climbs above the upper boundary, the kidneys filter out the excess and send it out of the body in your urine, thereby decreasing the concentration of sodium in the blood.

So far so good. However...

Salt and Blood Pressure. In a large number of people, a problem occurs: the kidneys don't do a good job of filtering out the excess. If you are one of these people and your sodium concentration is too high, your body must rely on a second mechanism: it must "dilute" the sodium.

It tries to do this by making you thirsty, and by drawing water out of other tissues. (One of the tissues it draws water from is the salivary glands, which dry up a bit, in turn drying your mouth; this contributes to your feeling of thirst.)

The extra fluid you drink and the extra fluid drawn from tissue increases the volume of blood in your blood vessels, which increases your blood pressure.

High blood pressure (**hypertension**) has no overt symptoms (hence the grisly nickname *the silent killer*). But prolonged high blood pressure damages the kidneys. High blood pressure also causes the heart to work harder than it should, increasing the risk of heart failure and heart attack.

The first line of treatment for high blood pressure is salt restriction.

Not everyone who has hypertension has **salt-sensitive hypertension**; that is, salt is not the bad guy in every case of high blood pressure. But it is in many, and salt restriction is a good non-drug approach to controlling hypertension.

What Specific Conditions are Caused By Too Much Salt?

Of particular interest to athletes is the fact that excess salt can cause muscular weakness, fatigue and cramping.

How Can I Avoid These Problems?

You can avoid these problems by simply eating less salt. Eat fewer processed foods—processed foods tend to contain much more salt than unprocessed foods. Also, look for low- or no-salt versions of popular foods. Specialty manufacturers are coming out with ever-increasing numbers of these more-healthful alternatives to traditionally salted items. These low-salt versions usually cost more than their salty counterparts. Why? Without added salt, processed foods taste quite bland. To make them taste better, the food processors are compelled to add more meat, vegetables, herbs, and spices—in other words, they have to add more food to their food. This is much more expensive (but much better for you) than covering up the blandness with a lot of salt.

Be aware that salt is not the only source of sodium. Many other additives used in food processing don't taste salty but contain a high dose of sodium. The table below will help you determine what adjustments to make in your selection of foods.

SALT CONTENT OF SELECTED FOODS

FOOD AND AMOUNT	MG. OF SODIUM (approx.)
Take-out Chicken Dinner (1)	1500
Dill Pickle (1 large)	1400
Cheese Pizza (1/2 of 12" pizza)	1350
Pancakes (3, from mix)	1150
Canned Chicken Noodle Soup (1 cup)	1100
Soy Sauce (1 tablespoon)	1000
Canned Tomato Soup (1 cup)	932
Egg McMuffin (1)	885
Take-out Fish & Chips Dinner (1)	840
Cheeseburger (1)	767
Oatmeal (1 cup)	523
Processed Cheese (1 ounce)	400
Barbecue Sauce (1 tablespoon)	300
Catsup (1 teaspoon)	181
Cheddar Cheese (1 ounce)	176
Egg (1)	159

The other adjustment to make is: stop cooking with salt, and stop adding salt to foods before you eat them.

Salt is an acquired taste. If you grow up eating salted foods, they taste bland to you unsalted. But that *changes* after you've been off salt for a while. A few weeks of eating low-salt foods is usually enough to temper your "salt tooth." You'll find you prefer the natural flavors of foods to the salt-masked flavors and don't miss the taste of salt in them.

The benefits of eating less salt are worth the effort it takes to become comfortable not eating as much.

- The average American eats *twenty to thirty times* as much salt as necessary for optimum health and physical performance.

- Excess salt causes serious problems such as hypertension, which can lead to kidney damage, heart disease and increased risk of stroke.

- Excess salt increases the tendency of muscles to cramp

- Guideline for optimum athletic nutrition:

  - Reduce salt intake by avoiding high salt foods, buying low- or no-salt alternatives, and not adding salt during cooking or eating.

SUGAR

Sugar has been the subject of a lot of controversy. Some of sugar's critics equate it with poison, yet some respected researchers say the criticisms are unfounded. Where lies the truth?

Two Sides to the Story

First, we should make clear that we're talking here about *refined* sugar—**sucrose**—like the sugar in a sugar bowl. We're not talking about complex carbohydrates, which are long strings of sugars.

Sugar's enemies say it causes all sorts of physical and even emotional problems. The long list includes claims that sugar causes or contributes to:

- glucose intolerance
- diabetes
- elevated cholesterol
- hypertension

- coronary artery disease
- behavior changes in both children and adults
- problems in the central nervous system
- obesity
- increased likelihood of developing gallstones
- lower bioavailability of vitamins and minerals
- dietary deficiencies
- cavities
- cancer

The Center for Food Safety and Applied Nutrition recently created a Sugar Task Force to look into all of these claims.

The task force reviewed the scientific research and concluded only one of these claims—the claim that sugar causes cavities—was based on conclusive scientific evidence. Their overall finding was that there is no conclusive evidence that sugar is a hazard to the public at the levels currently consumed.

Nevertheless, there is some preliminary evidence that sugar may indeed contribute to obesity (which in turn increases the risk of glucose intolerance and diabetes), lessen the likelihood of getting a balanced diet (leading to potential dietary deficiencies such as insufficient chromium), and increase blood triglyceride (fat) and cholesterol (increasing the risk of coronary artery disease).

So What Should I Think About Sugar?

What does sugar offer to your diet?

Calories. That's it. Beyond that, sugar has no nutritional value. Foodstuffs that offer concentrated calories but no other nutritional benefits—no vitamins, minerals, or fiber—are said to have **empty calories**.

If you consume many empty calories, one of two things has to happen: either you stick to your appropriate calorie intake and risk not getting all the nutrients you might otherwise get, or you eat enough additional calories to meet your nutritional needs while the empty calories carry you over the appropriate calorie limit.

Either way, sugar can only be a minus in your diet.

Even though some of the claims about sugar have not yet been conclusively born out, the preliminary findings mentioned are cause for concern. In light of these preliminary findings and the absence of nutritional benefits, it is reasonable to decrease consumption of refined sugar.

Is Table Sugar All I Have to Avoid?

Unfortunately, cutting down on sugar is not as simple as merely substituting with Sweet 'n' Lo in your morning coffee. Sugar comes in a variety of forms, and under a number of names. Many, many products contain far more sugar than you would expect.

In order to avoid sugar you have to recognize it, so let's go through some of its more common incarnations here.

Sucrose

Sucrose is the most common sugar you'll encounter. Sucrose is ordinary white table sugar, refined from sugar cane and sugar beets. As explained in Chapter 5, sucrose is a *disaccharide* made of two *monosaccharides*—glucose and fructose, linked together. Sucrose is the sugar found in brown sugar, powdered sugar, and turbinado sugar.

Corn Syrup

Corn syrup is also widely used, because it's inexpensive to produce. It is almost 100% glucose, made by treating corn starch with acid.

Glucose is two-thirds as sweet as sucrose, but has only half the calories (because glucose is a monosaccharide, and sucrose is a disaccharide). So corn syrup can provide an equal amount of sweetness for slightly fewer calories than sucrose.

Fructose

Fructose is *not* a sugar substitute, it is sugar—in spite of the *no sugar* labels on some products containing it. Fructose is also called "fruit sugar," because it is commonly found in fruit. Of all the sugars, fructose is most closely linked to increased cholesterol levels.

Fructose is about seventy percent sweeter than table sugar, but has only half the calories (as with glucose, because fructose is a monosaccharide, and sucrose is a disaccharide), so you can get the same amount of sweetness from fructose for considerably fewer calories than sucrose. This is the rationale behind advertising campaigns that fructose is "lower in calories" than table sugar. However, you only reap the "lower in calories" benefit if you use less.

Brown sugar is white sugar with a little molasses added back in for color and flavor. The darker the brown sugar, the more molasses has been added back in. Brown sugar holds no nutritional advantages over white sugar.

Brown Sugar

Raw sugar is what cane becomes after the first in a long series of steps in the processing, refining, and packaging sequence. The United States Department of Agriculture states that raw sugar is "unfit for direct use as a food ingredient because of the impurities it ordinarily contains." Raw sugar should not be confused with **turbinado sugar**. It is illegal to sell raw sugar in the United States.

Raw Sugar

Turbinado sugar is partially refined. It is refined enough to remove the impurities that the USDA says make raw sugar "unfit for direct use as a food ingredient" but is not refined to the point of removing the molasses. It is the molasses, in fact, that gives turbinado sugar its light brown color.

Other than that, it is identical to table sugar. Turbinado manufacturers try to associate their product with "raw, natural sugar" by giving it names containing the word *Raw* and producing it in big, coarse crystals, but it is far from being the natural, unrefined product the names imply. It actually goes through almost the same entire refining process that white sugar goes through. The incremental difference in "naturalness" is meaningless.

Turbinado Sugar

Powdered sugar, also called **confectioners' sugar** or **icing sugar**, is simply plain white sugar in powdered form. A small amount of cornstarch is usually added to the product to reduce lumping.

Powdered Sugar

Invert sugar is not something you can buy, but it is something you see from time to time on ingredient lists. Invert sugar is

Invert Sugar

regular table sugar, the disaccharide *sucrose*, chemically split into its two component monosaccharides, *glucose* and *fructose*.

Maple Sugar

Maple syrup, in its pure form, is mostly sucrose, with some invert sugar. Most maple syrup sold in supermarkets is imitation maple syrup.

In its impure form—which is more common—true maple syrup sometimes contains a chemical called *paraformaldehyde* along with the sugar. This chemical is used to make the sap in maple trees run faster, and is not particularly good for you.

Molasses

Molasses is a byproduct of sugar processing. It is the dark liquid that remains after the sucrose crystals are removed from sugar cane or beet juice. There are three kinds: **unsulfured** (light and dark), **sulfured** (light and dark), and **blackstrap**.

Unsulfured molasses is made from sun-ripened sugar cane grown specifically for molasses-making. Sulfured molasses is so-called because it retains sulfur from the sulfur fumes used in manufacturing sugar. Whether *light* or *dark* depends on the point during the sugar- making process the molasses came from.

Sugar cane juice is boiled several times during the process of extracting sugar. The residue from the first boiling is called **light molasses**. The residue from the second boiling is called **dark molasses**. The residue from the third boiling is called **blackstrap molasses**.

The darker the molasses, the better nutritionally. Blackstrap molasses contains small but not insignificant amounts of calcium, iron, potassium, and B vitamins. The presence of these minerals makes blackstrap molasses slightly more nutritious than table sugar, but not enough to put it on the recommended eating list. If you are going to use a sweetener, dark molasses is nutritionally your best choice.

Honey

Honey is a liquid mixture of fructose, glucose, and water. Advocates of honey point to its "naturalness," the fact it doesn't need refining, and that it contains potassium, calcium, a few trace elements, a few B vitamins, some enzymes and some amino acids.

Detractors point out honey rots teeth faster than table sugar, that some honeys contain cancer-causing chemicals bees pick up from flowers, and that honey may cause the frequently-fatal food poisoning **botulism** in infants. (Indeed, pediatricians recommend that *no* infant be given honey.)

The potassium and other nutrients found in honey are present in such tiny amounts that, from a nutritional standpoint, they are insignificant. Consumers Union has calculated that you would have to eat 200 tablespoons (12.5 cups, over *nine pounds*) of honey to meet your daily requirement of calcium.

There is no scientific evidence honey is any better, or any less bad, for you than table sugar.

Incidentally, in light of this, where do honeys that are *raw, unfiltered, unheated,* or *unpasteurized* stand? They are likely to have more bacterial contamination but are no better nutritionally.

Now that you've met sugar in its various disguises, you're ready to approach the labels on processed foods. Pre-sweetened breakfast cereals are the major offenders in the hidden-sugar category. Some of them are over *fifty percent sugar!*

Be aware that manufacturers are required by law to list ingredients on the label in their order of prominence by weight. Take a look at the grocery store at some popular cereals, and note how many list sugar as the *first* ingredient!

Some athletes use processed foods high in simple sugars as a concentrated form of calories. But complex carbohydrates have just as many calories as simple carbohydrates, and they are much better for you. As mentioned in Chapter 5, the American Dietetic Association recommends athletes get from sixty to sixty-five percent of all calories from carbohydrates (sixty-five to seventy percent for endurance athletes), with not more than ten percent from simple carbohydrates.

As with salt, a sweet tooth is an acquired taste. With a few simple steps over a few weeks' time, you can greatly lessen your craving for sugar.

Don't drink soft drinks! Soft drinks have an incredible amount of sugar in them, and because they are so sweet, they do a terrible job of quenching thirst.

Step #1

If you are like most Americans, you drink at least one soft drink a day, so there's room for some real progress here. This doesn't mean you should never have another soft drink for the rest of your life. It just means you should make a conscious effort to cut down on soft drink consumption. (Adolescent males consume an average of over a half-pound of sugar *a day*, much of that from soft drinks.)

Nor does this mean you should drink diet soda instead. The sweeteners in diet soft drinks—**aspartame** (Nutrasweet) and **saccharin**—may be just fine for you. Then again, they may not. Saccharin has already been demonstrated to cause bladder cancer in laboratory mice (admittedly in whopping doses). The jury is still out, so it's a good idea to avoid sugar substitutes.

Substituting milk or fruit juice is a good way to get extra nutrients where you were getting only empty calories before. This is especially important for teen-aged women, who get far too much phosphate (abundant in soft drinks) and far too little calcium (abundant in milk).

Step #2

If you eat those obscenely sweet kiddies' breakfast cereals, stop! You may as well dump a quarter-cup of sugar and a quarter-cup of white flour in your breakfast bowl and pour on the milk. Not that the "natural"-appearing cereals are that much better. Many granolas are around thirty percent sugar. Read the labels, and find a cereal that you like that doesn't have more sugar than cereal.

Step #3

Shy away from the sugar bowl. Especially at breakfast! Most people habitually put the same number of teaspoons of sugar on their cereal and in their coffee—even on their grapefuit. Break the habit. Cut back a bit; you can get by with less sugar than you think. Also, less of a sugar load in the morning may make you less susceptible to a mid-morning slump.

Step #4

Eat smaller portions of the sweet things you do eat. If you feel like having *just a little something sweet*, have a 0.16-oz. Hershey's Kiss (25 calories) instead of a 1.65-oz. Hershey Bar (250 calories). Have a third of a piece of pecan pie instead of the whole thing. One scoop of Häagen Dazs will do just as well as two.

Eat more fresh fruit. An apple has fewer calories, more nutrients and fiber, fills you up more and keeps you satisfied longer than a candy bar.

Step #5

■ **Aside from calories, sugar has no nutritional value.**

■ **Many claims have been made about sugar causing physical and emotional problems, but not all of these have been substantiated by research. However...**

❑ **high sugar consumption clearly results in an increased risk of cavities**

❑ **preliminary evidence suggests that sugar may contribute to obesity, which in turn increases the risk of glucose intolerance and diabetes; lessen the likelihood of getting a balanced diet, leading to potential dietary deficiencies such as insufficient chromium; and increase blood triglyceride (fat) and cholesterol, increasing the risk of coronary artery disease.**

■ **Guideline for optimum athletic nutrition:**

❑ **In light of the evidence cited above and sugar's lack of nutritional value, it would seem prudent to keep sugar consumption to a minimum.**

❖   ❖   ❖

PART THREE

BAD NUTRITION

Before examining optimal sports nutrition, we're going to examine some less-than-optimal sports nutrition as practiced by many athletes.

The purpose of this investigation is not to criticize or belittle anyone, but rather to expose the nutritional pitfalls into which the unwary may fall.

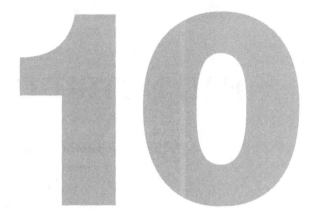

UNSUPPORTED CLAIMS: SEPARATING THE FRAUD FROM THE FRINGE

Nutrition is a complicated and often perplexing field. Experts frequently disagree, even on basic points. In fact, it isn't always clear who *is* an expert, and who's not.

A certain amount of information is generally accepted as fact—borne out by experience and by relatively well-understood laws of biochemistry. Beyond this, though, lies a great grey region of undocumented products and practices, supported only by logical hypothesis, folk tradition, or the fervent testimonies of a few loyal users.

Our purpose is to keep you from getting lost in this relatively uncharted area. To do this we've tried to make a basic distinction between nutritional claims and practices which can be shown to be invalid—even fraudulent—and those which are simply unsupported by scientific evidence to date.

NUTRITIONAL QUACKERY— AN OVERVIEW

Nutritional quackery—the peddling of bogus nutrition-related products and services—is big business. The House Subcommittee on Health and Long-term Care estimates quackery is a ten-billion dollar a year business, and growing fast. There are several reasons this is so.

Enforcing laws against health fraud are the responsibility of the United States Food and Drug Administration (FDA). However, the FDA's priorities are (1) supervision of prescription drugs and (2) food safety. The one-half of one percent of its budget the FDA currently allots for fighting quackery is spent mostly on efforts to educate the public against getting taken in. The FDA has prosecuted only two criminal actions involving fraudulent nutritional supplements in the past twenty-two years.

In this environment, nutritional quacks operate freely and openly, knowing their bogus claims will not land them in jail.

In addition, the public's interest in health and fitness has grown dramatically in the last fifteen years. More people are exercising and watching their diets than ever before. The prevailing standards of attractiveness are centered on leanness, fitness, and energy. People of all ages want to look better, play harder, and live longer. So even if the nutritional quacks weren't coming out in greater numbers—as they most assuredly are—their businesses would be growing just because more people are interested in what they purport to offer.

Finally, and most important, people *want to believe.*

Wouldn't it be great if you could take a pill that would make you "burn fat faster" so you could eat anything you desired without gaining unwanted weight? Sure it would. And if you saw such pills advertised, would you think they'd really work? Probably not. But if you found it very hard to keep your weight down, and the pills only cost a dollar a day to take, you very well might buy them. Anyone might. Even though we know better, we will often pay good money for the chance that the impossible will happen.

Athletes are particularly susceptible to nutritional quackery. Serious competitive athletes, especially, live in an environment in which the smallest advantage can make the difference between winning and losing.

People are hurt by nutritional quackery in at least three ways.

- They are sometimes directly hurt by the products or services themselves.

- They are sometimes hurt when their reliance on bogus products or services prevents them from seeking available effective treatments for their problems

- They are hurt by wasting their money, often in surprisingly large amounts. Nutritional quacks know that more expensive products and services will be perceived as more effective.

SUSPECT INDUSTRY PRACTICES

First Amendment Protection for Bogus Claims

Probably the single biggest ripoff in the nutrition industry is the practice of selling nutritional supplements for which bogus claims are made. Often the claim is that the product will treat or prevent a particular disease. Sometimes the claim is that the product will slow aging. Other times it is that the product will increase energy or general well-being. For athletes, the claims are for increased strength, increased muscle mass, improved reaction times, decreased recovery times, greater speed, agility, and on and on.

These claims are often made in the absence of any scientific evidence. The manufacturers count on the buyer wanting to believe the product will work.

Read the labels carefully. The claims do *not* appear on the labels of the products. Instead, the claims are made in pamphlets which are close by; in books available for perusal; in the flyers that get put in your bag when you're checking out; in nutrition articles written by the same people who sell the products; or in nutrition articles written by business associates of the people who sell the products.

Why do all these claims appear elsewhere but not on the bottle?

Unsupported claims cannot legally appear on the label of the bottle, because that falls under the jurisdiction of the FDA, and it is a violation of FDA laws.

Unsupported claims *can*, however, be published in pamphlets, books, flyers, and magazine articles, because these claims, no matter how false, are protected by the First Amendment. They needn't contain a particle of truth, and often they don't. You could, if you wanted to, sell bottles of Big Buff pills, alongside a flyer that said *Iron Curtain Researchers Prove Big Buff Pills Give You 36" Biceps Overnight*.

As long as the bottle label displayed an innocuous statement like *Nutritional Supplement for Bodybuilders*, and nothing else, you would be operating entirely within the law.

If the claims are true and verifiable, you can bet the manufacturers will be trumpeting that fact at every opportunity, including on the label. So read the labels! If they don't say what you have been led to believe about the product, what you have been led to believe may not be supportable.

Drugs as Food

The labels on nutritional products invariably state that the products are "dietary supplements"—in other words, food.

This is also grounds for suspicion. The manufacturers and distributors of nutritional supplements do not want their products to be subject to the FDA regulations governing *drugs*, which are much more stringent than regulations governing *food*. Under the law, a product is a drug if it is "intended for use in the diagnosis, cure, mitigation, treatment or prevention of disease in man or other animals." The consequence of a product being classified as a drug is that it can only be legally marketed if it has FDA approval or is "generally recognized as safe and effective."

Companies marketing products whose safety and effectiveness have not been well-established do not want to subject themselves to this kind of restriction. By labeling their products as food supplements, and making their claims elsewhere, the companies can market a product which does not have to be "generally recognized as safe and effective." As long as their products do not contain controlled or restricted substances, the FDA generally lets them operate in this way.

It is important to recognize that this distinction between food and drug is a hazy one, and not all products labeled as foods are benign. Some contain potentially harmful substances, and some can even be fatal to individuals sensitive to them.

Multilevel Marketing Schemes

Multilevel marketing organizations are basically pyramid schemes, which lure people to become distributors of their products by convincing them they'll become rich in the process.

These schemes create small armies of people who believe that their one chance to get rich depends on selling you their line of products. As a result, they have a powerful incentive to make all sorts of exaggerated claims about what those products will do. They also have an even more powerful incentive to encourage the distributors working below them to make such claims. Some of the most outrageous claims come out of these organizations.

Diagnostic Tests

An increasingly popular form of nutritional quackery is the offering of tests to evaluate individuals' nutritional status. Not only are most of these tests invalid, they also tend to be expensive, and are often followed by "prescriptions"—and sometimes direct sales—of products to fill the client's purported nutritional "needs." The most widely used tests include:

Hair Analysis

This test is just what it sounds like. A sample of your hair is analyzed in an attempt to determine the status of various minerals in your body.

Although hair analysis is useful in the fields of epidemiology and forensic medicine in assessing heavy metal poisoning (e.g. poisoning by lead or mercury), it is *useless* for individual nutritional guidance. For most minerals, no correlation has been established between amount in hair and nutritional status. Furthermore, mineral content of hair varies greatly depending on the kind of shampoo used, coloring or bleaching, age, geographic location, and hair growth rate. Lack of consistent test results is also a problem: studies have demonstrated enormous variation from lab to lab and even within the same lab for test results from identical samples.

Cytotoxic Testing For Allergies

This test (sometimes called **leukocytotoxic testing**) has been around for over thirty years, but has become popular only recently. It is based on the premise that if you take a sample of someone's blood and expose it to the dried extracts of various foods, you can spot the person's allergies by the way the white blood cells react.

Does it work? Both the American Academy of Allergy and Immunology and the National Institute of Allergy and Infectious Disease consider cytotoxic testing invalid and of no clinical use. A National Institute of Health publication states cytotoxic testing "has not been proved to be effective," and that results "have not been shown to be reliable and reproducible in controlled studies."

Computerized Dietary Questionnaires

The idea here is that you answer *yes* or *no* to several hundred questions (for example, *Do you catch cold easily?*), and the computer analyzes your answers and gives you an elaborate and impressive-looking printout telling you your nutritional status.

On the surface that sounds plausible, but the flaw is summed up in a saying familiar to all computer programmers: garbage in, garbage out. In other words, the computer's analysis is only as good as the information it has to work with. With these tests, that information is usually not very good. The tests invariably diagnose nutritional deficiencies, because they're intended to encourage the sale of nutritional products. They're about as personalized and accurate as your daily horoscope in the newspaper.

There *are* legitimate computerized dietary assessment plans, but they differ from those described above in that the legitimate ones require considerable dietary specificity. It is not possible for a questionnaire to evaluate dietary nutritional shortcomings unless it asks for a list of absolutely everything you have eaten for at least several days. Nor is it possible for a questionnaire to *diagnose* nutritional deficiencies based on vague questions such as *Do you catch cold easily?*

Urinary Amino Acid Tests

This involves submitting a sample of urine to be analyzed for the presence of amino acids. On the basis of which amino acids are found and in what quantities, the conductor of the test recommends what kind of amino acid supplements the athlete should take.

Again, it sounds plausible. Only one problem: *amino acids don't show up in the urine.* Unless you have kidney disease, which few athletes have, your kidneys don't excrete amino acids in the urine. It's like analyzing your car's exhaust to determine what's in the glove compartment.

Diagnosis of Deficiency Symptoms

Let's take a little test. Answer yes or no to the following questions:

Do you ever feel a little tired, maybe in the afternoon after lunch?
Do you ever lose your appetite?
Do you ever feel a little irritable or depressed?
Do you ever have trouble falling asleep?
Do you ever have little aches or pains?
Do you ever have skin problems?

Do you ever have indigestion, constipation, or diarrhea?
Do you ever have headaches?
Do you ever feel a little nauseated?
Do your eyes ever itch or burn?

If you answered *yes* to any of the ten questions, you show some signs of deficiency of one or more of the following nutrients: Vitamin A, Vitamin B1, Vitamin B2, Vitamin B3, Vitamin B6, Vitamin B12, pantothenic acid, biotin, folic acid, Vitamin C, Vitamin D, Vitamin E. That is, you do if you are susceptible to this form of nutritional quackery.

Obviously, most people would answer *yes* to most if not all of the ten questions above. Do most people suffer from the deficiencies just mentioned? No.

Nutritionists who diagnose your "deficiencies" according to your "symptoms"—and who invariably stand ready to sell you supplements to correct those "deficiencies"—are misrepresenting a fundamental fact: deficiency symptoms don't show up unless the deficiency is *severe*. Mild deficiencies don't produce those symptoms.

Seldom do people's diets—even bad diets—provide them with less than 70% of the recommended daily allowances (the RDA's) of the various nutrients. Furthermore, the RDA's are calculated to provide a *safety margin*—that is, quite a bit more of each nutrient than we actually need to avoid a deficiency. Very seldom do Americans suffer anything more than very mild deficiencies—certainly much too mild to be producing deficiency symptoms.

A genuine Vitamin B1 deficiency *will* make you tired and irritable. But if you're tired and irritable, does that necessarily mean you have a Vitamin B1 deficiency? No. Everybody gets tired and irritable. A Vitamin B1 deficiency is a very unlikely cause of it. But this backwards reasoning is the basis for selling a lot of vitamin and mineral supplements.

Other Dubious Tests

Nutritional experts consider a number of other so-called diagnostic tests to be of questionable value. These include: **LivCell testing** (involving a video camera and a darkfield microscope to detect diseases); **Ream's Test** (a kind of saliva analysis); and **Applied Kinesiology** (which tests muscles for strength or weakness while the person is in contact with various foods and other substances).

This discussion might lead one to ask: *Is there a good test that will determine my overall nutritional status?* The answer is: *No.*

NUTRITIONAL PRODUCT EVALUATION

Here's a look at a few examples of claims for specific products. Some of these products have been shown to be ineffective, for others there is no information for or against. The list is far from exhaustive, but should help you decide whether you want to invest the time and money to pursue the results these products promise to deliver.

Bioflavinoids

THE CLAIMS: Many claims are made for bioflavinoids, including that bioflavinoids are good for herpes, make you bruise less easily, reduce your risk of atherosclerosis, protect against arthritis, reduce inflammation, and decrease menopausal symptoms.

THE FACTS: The bioflavinoids are actually a group of over 200 compounds found in many plants. At one time they were collectively called **Vitamin P**, but that label was dropped when scientists determined that the bioflavinoids are *not* essential to man or animals.

There is no RDA for bioflavinoids, and it is very likely there is no such thing as a bioflavinoid deficiency. No risks have been associated with taking bioflavinoids, but *no benefits have been documented.* The possibility of toxic side-effects from long-term excessive use has not been ruled out.

Blue-Green Algae

THE CLAIMS: Blue-green algae is touted as a cure for, among other things, herpes, arthritis, leprosy, allergies, Alzheimer's disease, sickle cell anemia, and anorexia nervosa.

THE FACTS: There is no evidence to support the claims made for the various products derived from this substance.

Although the algae is advertised as being free of impurities, an FDA laboratory analysis of one such product turned up parts of flies, maggots, ants, ticks, and a host of other unwelcome ingredients.

Carnitine

THE CLAIMS: The most common claim about carnitine is that it is a "fat burner"—that it increases your body's ability to utilize fat for energy during exercise. Additional claims are made that carnitine boosts energy, prevents injury, and even prevents heart disease.

THE FACTS: Carnitine facilitates the transport of fatty acids across the mitochondrial membrane—a process critically important to fat utilization and energy production. A severe carnitine deficiency may in fact interfere with fat utilization.

However, scientists have looked closely at the relationship of carnitine metabolism and exercise, and have concluded that a normal diet provides tissue carnitine levels entirely adequate to support fat utilization during exercise. Considerable evidence bears out that supplemental carnitine does not enhance the process.

Garlic

THE CLAIMS: Claims for garlic date back thousands of years. Most common among them is the belief that garlic will cure hay fever, arthritis, sleeping problems, lung problems, tuberculosis, athlete's foot, digestive problems, and heart disease, and that it will cleanse the blood and retard aging.

THE FACTS: There is no evidence garlic will do the more exotic things claimed for it. However, it does have certain good qualities: it may may have a positive effect on cholesterol; it may also help dissolve blood clots and keep clots from forming. Some preliminary work even suggests it may protect against cancer in laboratory animals.

In large doses, garlic can cause stomach damage, so don't megadose if you take garlic supplements.

Glandular Concentrates

THE CLAIMS: The basic claim is that if you ingest a "raw gland concentrate"—that is, a tissue concentrate from the organ or gland of an animal—it will heal or help build that same organ or gland within your body.

THE FACTS: This goes back to the ancient belief that if you eat the flesh of an animal, you take on the characteristics of that animal. These concentrates are available, at last count, for the following glands and organs: adrenals, thyroid, thymus, pancreas, pituitary, liver, brain, stomach, lung, heart, spleen, kidney, testes, and ovaries.

Having read the chapter on Protein, you can easily predict what will happen to glandular concentrates. They will be treated just like any other protein—shredded in the stomach and small intestine, and absorbed as single amino acids and short chains two or three amino acids long. By the time they are absorbed these glandular concentrates bear absolutely no resemblance to the glands they came from. Furthermore, glandular concentrates are usually prepared at low temperatures, and as a result often contain unacceptably high levels of bacteria—making them potentially hazardous to your health.

Herbal Weight Loss Products

THE CLAIMS: These products claim to help you lose weight quickly.

THE FACTS: Many of these products contain ingredients that act as laxatives. One successfully marketed "natural herbal" weight loss product contains substantial doses of cascara, a powerful laxative made from a dried bark. And indeed, it does cause weight loss, as diarrhea often does. Taking laxatives on a regular basis can cause a dependency on them, as well as a deficiency in potassium and magnesium.

You should be careful when dealing with herbs in general. The fact that something is *herbal* does not mean it is necessarily harmless. Some herbs are quite powerful, and some may contain toxic chemicals. After all, cyanide, poison hemlock, and deadly nightshade are all herbal substances.

Oral Chelation

THE CLAIMS: The claim is that oral chelation fights heart disease by removing the calcium in the plaque that builds up on artery walls.

THE FACTS: Oral chelation is a descendant of intravenous chelation therapy—a heart disease treatment which is itself unproven.

In the intravenous version, a chemical called EDTA is injected into the bloodstream, supposedly to unclog vessels in the heart. This therapy does not have FDA approval, has never been shown to be effective, and may cause kidney damage.

Oral chelation products are mixtures of vitamins, minerals, amino acids, and (usually) EDTA, sold for the purpose of treatment or prevention of "clogged blood vessels." Oral chelation products are illegal. Nonetheless, it is still possible to buy them from mail order companies, health food stores, and door-to-door salespeople. The FDA considers oral chelation therapy to be a form of health fraud, and has begun a nationwide effort to remove oral chelation products from the market.

PABA

THE CLAIMS: Promoters of PABA (para-aminobenzoic acid) claim that orally ingesting this substance will promote growth, cure infertility and impotence, and darken greying hair.

THE FACTS: PABA makes a good sunscreen, and is used topically in suntan lotions for this purpose. There is no evidence that oral ingestion of PABA has any nutritional significance, although it may cause nausea and vomiting.

Royal Jelly and Bee Pollen

THE CLAIMS: The claim is that these bee products will increase fertility, longevity, endurance and strength, and will help the body defend against stress.

THE FACTS: Neither of these substances is bad for you. They are high in B vitamins, and contain a number of other nutrients. However, the claims for them are unsubstantiated. There is no reason to believe they will confer any benefits beyond those available from a normal balanced intake of nutrients.

Seaweed

THE CLAIMS: Seaweed is claimed to be a rich source of protein, to be effective in treating spastic colitis, constipation, hypoglycemia, hypercholesterolemia, and hay fever, and to be helpful in dieting.

THE FACTS: Seaweed, or kelp, is a rich source of iodine. Virtually every kelp tablet available will provide the RDA of 150 micrograms. Beyond that, no beneficial effects have been scientifically established. Seaweed is only 6% protein, and the protein is of low quality.

Superoxide Dismutase (SOD) Dismutase;

THE CLAIMS: The claim is that SOD tablets will make you live longer.

THE FACTS: Superoxide dismutase is an enzyme. Along with vitamins E and C and a few other antioxidant substances, it helps take care of free radicals which, though a normal byproduct of your body's metabolism, could otherwise damage your cells and advance the aging process. SOD tablets are marketed on the theory that if a normal production of antioxidants is good, extra ones must be better.

Remember, *all enzymes are proteins*. And like any other protein, SOD is shredded in the stomach and small intestines and is absorbed as single amino acids and short chains two or three amino acids long, which bear no resemblance whatsoever to the original protein.

The studies done so far provide no evidence that SOD supplements prolong your life span.

WHEN TO BE SUSPICIOUS

Here's a five-step approach to evaluating nutritional claims:

First, consider the nature of the claim being made.

As the saying goes, if it sounds too good to be true, it probably is. Some quacks have no shame, and seemingly will make *any* claim, no matter how preposterous, if they think enough people will go for it. Often they promise help that *nobody* can deliver. Include in this category products that promise increased sex drive or sexual potency; miracle cures for cancer, AIDS, and other diseases; fast and easy weight loss; risk-free sex; restored youth or slower aging; longer life. Ask yourself whether it's even reasonably *possible* for this claim to be true.

Beware of ambiguous claims. Some claims are so vague you could never really tell whether the product lived up to them or not.

Include here products that promise to do things such as strengthen the heart; improve circulation; regenerate cells; purify the blood; improve mental functioning; strengthen the immune system; strengthen the liver; protect against the aging process; neutralize poisons; cleanse your body of "toxins"; improve skin and hair; improve digestion. When you consider such a claim, try and figure out just what you'd expect to see or feel happen if the product worked. If you find the answer elusive, you have reason to be suspicious. In general, be wary of products that promise to "protect," "strengthen," "purify," or "prevent" *anything*.

Second, look at who is making the claim. Look for legitimate credentials, degrees, and institutional affiliations. Beware of anyone presenting himself or herself as simply a "consultant"; beware of anyone listing a degree such as Ph.D. without listing the school, or of anyone whose only affiliation is with an institute or university started by them.

Third, look at what kind of evidence is being offered to support the claim. Is the claim supported by controlled scientific studies, or is it based only on anecdotal evidence?

Hard scientific findings are obviously the best support for a nutritional claim. If the claim is supported only by personal endorsements, you can bet no scientific evidence exists. That doesn't mean the claim is necessarily bogus—every new idea is unsupported until it has been researched—but it is a factor to weigh.

Fourth, look at who stands to make money from the claim. Think of where the money will go if you buy the product. The closer it will go to the source of the claim, the more reason you have to be suspicious. On the other hand, if the person making the claim does not stand to benefit from your purchase, he or she is more likely to be credible.

Fifth, look at how much the product or service costs. In general, though not always, the more expensive a nutritional product is, the more reason you have to be suspicious. Good nutrition is simply not an expensive proposition.

In making their products expensive, manufacturers take advantage of a basic fact of human nature: something that costs more is perceived to be worth more. Try to determine objectively if what you're buying is fairly priced for what it is.

■ Today, hundreds of products promise rapid weight loss, muscle gain, long life and freedom from disease. The fact is few of these claims are supported by hard scientific evidence. In this chapter, we've explored some common claims and nutritional practices which, to a greater or lesser degree, seem to warrant caution on the part of the athlete.

■ Admittedly, the existence or lack of scientific evidence is not a foolproof standard by which to evaluate a claim—often no evidence exists only because no research has been done. Still, the scientific method, in which results are measurable and reproducible, is the only objective yardstick we have. Beyond this, you must supplement your training with healthy doses of common sense.

❖   ❖   ❖

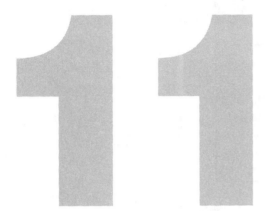

BAD EATING

If you've been reading straight through from the beginning of the book, by now you should have a pretty good idea of what *good eating* means. We'll get more specific later on. For now, suffice it to say the guidelines include:

- each day consuming roughly the number of calories you need to meet your body's energy demands
- getting most of those calories from complex carbohydrates, and smaller proportions from fat and protein
- eating a variety of fresh foods to ensure a balanced intake of vitamins and minerals
- not consuming things that are bad for you
- not consuming *too much* of things that are good for you

Good eating is just about that simple! (Only in the quest for peak athletic performance do you stand to benefit from a more exacting approach.)

Since sound nutrition can, for most purposes, be achieved by following those few simple guidelines, you would think it would be the rule and bad eating the exception.

Unfortunately, that's not the case. A number of forces conspire to make us eat badly. Cultural and social forces in particular play significant roles.

Different ethnic backgrounds bring with them particular eating habits—some good, some bad. Current popular culture, although idealizing the image of health and fitness, bombards us with products and advertising designed to lead us nutritionally astray. Our history still haunts us: many of today's eating habits are carry-overs from earlier times, when people led lives quite different from ours.

Also, we are just not taught to be nutrition-conscious. Basic nutrition classes are required in some schools, but they're not a high priority—schools have their hands full trying to make sure people can read and write.

Learning good nutrition is like learning any other skill— knowing what *not* to do is just as important as knowing what *to* do.

Even recognizing that each person is unique, and that each person's habits and daily life are a little different, we can make a number of observations about the nutritional quality of the typical American diet. It is:

- too high in calories
- too high in protein
- too high in fat
- too low in complex carbohydrates, but high in the nutritionally inferior simple carbs.
- too low in fiber
- exceptionally high in salt
- too high in sugar

Also, it creates mineral imbalances. One example: the typical high intake of phosphorus and low intake of calcium creates an imbalance that can lead to osteoporosis (loss of calcium from the bones), bad teeth, and aching muscles and bones.

The problems with this diet are more a matter of excesses than deficiencies. The result of those excesses—decreased physical efficiency and increased vulnerability to disease.

THE TYPICAL AMERICAN DIET

Given the typical American diet, it's no surprise that a great many Americans want to lose weight. It's also no surprise that a great deal of money is made selling useless and some-

FAD DIETS

times dangerous weight loss programs. Let's separate the good from the bad.

What qualifies a diet as a fad diet? Fad diets have two major characteristics:

- they promise rapid and permanent weight loss
- they purport to be based on some new principle or substance

Each of these characteristics provides a tip-off why fad diets don't work.

First, rapid weight loss is not only unhealthy, it's ineffective. What you want to lose is **fat**; what you lose *rapidly* is **water** and **muscle**.

The only way to lose fat and keep it off is to lose it *gradually*, by exercising and following a diet that keeps you adequately nourished, creates the calorie deficit required to stimulate fat metabolism, and becomes a part of your normal lifestyle.

Second, the claim that the diet is based on a new principle or substance should sound the quackery alarm loud and clear. The likelihood someone will discover a way to bypass the natural physical processes governing weight loss is essentially non-existent.

Before looking at some diets that have been popular in recent years, let's consider what criteria we would expect a *good* diet to meet. It should:

- be medically **safe**—no extremes
- be **gradual**—the loss should not exceed about two pounds per week
- provide **adequate nutrition**
- fit **comfortably** into the dieter's life
- encourage a **healthy lifestyle** that will allow the dieter to **keep the weight off**

None of the fad diets discussed below meet these criteria. Some are truly unsafe. Virtually none endorse gradual weight loss. Many are nutritionally inadequate. Few promote a lifestyle that will keep the weight off.

Fad diets come in three general types: (1) diets based on changing **macronutrient* intake; (2) diets based on accelerating fat metabolism; and (3) diets based on specific food combinations**. Here is a sampling of diets from each category.

The diets in this category promise you will lose weight and keep it off by changing the relative amounts of protein, carbohydrates, and fats you eat each day (as compared to the proportions believed today to be optimum: fifty-five to sixty percent carbohydrates, ten to fifteen percent protein, and twenty to thirty percent fat). This group includes, but is by no means limited to, the following:

The Caveman Diet. This diet is just what it sounds like—according to it, you should eat as the cavemen ate. Presumably you can still use silverware if you choose, but on this diet you eat primarily meat, fish, vegetables and fruit, and very few grains or dairy products.

Following the Caveman diet, you would consume more protein and less carbohydrate than current standards suggest. The primary flaws in this diet are:

- you would get too little calcium
- you would get too much fat (meat from modern domestic animals contains much more fat than meat from the wild animals of the paleolithic age)

Dr. Atkins' Diet Revolution. The revolution is a high-protein, high-fat, low-carbohydrate regimen in which calories are not restricted, under the assumption that only carbohydrates are responsible for gains in body fat (not true). Following this diet, you run the risk of becoming **ketotic**—that is, having an abnormally high number of ketones in blood and urine, a condition that can be fatal. You also run the risk of dehydration and calcium depletion, and take in a lot of saturated fat and cholesterol.

Incidently, high protein diets often start off with impressive and initially encouraging weight losses. That's because excess protein is a diuretic, making your kidneys put out a lot of water to flush out the excess urea. You *do* lose weight, but it is water weight, not fat weight.

---

*Macronutrients are those dietary components that have calories—namely fats, proteins, and carbohydrates. Nothing else you eat (vitamins, minerals, water) has any calories.

Fad Diets On Parade

Diets based on changing macronutrient intake

Zen Macrobiotics. This diet represents philosophy run amok. It separates foods into two groups—the yin and the yang. All modern illnesses, the belief goes, stem from an imbalance—too much yin or too much yang. The diet progresses in increasingly-restrictive stages, culminating in a regimen of only brown rice and herbal tea.

In its early stages, which amount to vegetarianism, the macrobiotic diet is actually rather healthful. However, the later stages shift the balance radically in favor of carbohydrates, and drastically reduce the intake of essential fats, protein, vitamins, and minerals. On this diet you can lose more than weight—longtime followers have suffered from severe malnutrition, and several have died.

Diets based on accelerating fat metabolism

"Fat burner diets" usually focus on one or more specific substances, and base their claims on the notion that these substances will help your body "burn" fat faster.

There is really no such thing as *burning fat* despite what a lot of advertisements would have you to believe. Fat, as explained in Chapter 6, is simply a long-term storage form of energy. Only by increasing the amount of energy you expend (or decreasing the amount of energy [calories] you take in) can you reduce the amount of fat you carry around. And the only way to do that is by exercising and restricting caloric intake. Although phrases such as *Melt fat off your body while you sleep!* certainly sound appealing, they are not based in reality.

Some of the more ingenious creations fall in this category, including:

The Grapefruit Diet. On this diet, you either eat grapefruit or drink grapefruit juice with every meal. The meals themselves are high-protein, high-fat, and low-carbohydrate—the exact opposite of what you should be eating. The theory here is that the grapefruit makes fat burn faster; however, there is nothing magical about a grapefruit that would cause this to happen. The diet is also high in saturated fat and cholesterol.

The Immune Power Diet. This highly creative work of fiction manages to weave weight loss, cytotoxic testing, and the fear of AIDS into one ambitious and completely baseless presentation.

The regimen progresses in three steps: first, identify food allergies and eliminate the foods indicated; second, lose weight to break the "immune-fat connection" (whatever that is); third, "rebuild" the immune system by taking an assortment of supplements.

Recall from the last chapter that cytotoxic allergy testing—recommended by this diet's author— is expensive and probably useless. The other flaws in this theory are that (1) only severe, chronic malnutrition—seldom seen in this country—will impair the immune system, and (2) no scientific evidence supports the idea that particular foods or supplements will either help *or* harm the immune system.

The Lecithin, B6, Apple Cider Vinegar, and Kelp Diet. The food part of this diet is low-fat and low-calorie, but the real interest comes from the theory based on the four ingredients named in the diet's title. The idea is that the kelp— by supplying iodine—will stimulate the thyroid gland while Vitamin B6 stimulates the burning of fat. The vinegar adds potassium and the lecithin emulsifies the whole mixture with the fat.

Nothing here is particularly unhealthy—it's just that iodine doesn't stimulate the thyroid gland (unless an iodine deficiency is present), Vitamin B6 doesn't stimulate the burning of fat, vinegar is a poor source of potassium, and there's no need to emulsify the mixture. Taken together, these ingredients don't do anything for weight loss that watching fat and calories wouldn't do by themselves.

Diets based on specific food combinations

The proponents of diets in this final category would have you believe they have elevated food combining to a high art—that they have hit upon that elusive combination of dishes that will make fat disappear quickly and easily. Unfortunately, it's just not that simple.

Our samples here include:

The Beverly Hills Diet. This diet is built on the idea that undigested food is what turns to body fat. The diet emphasizes a combination of specific fruits, on the premise that the enzymes in these fruits can digest the undigested food remaining in our gastrointestinal tracts—thereby preventing it from turning to fat.

Several problems here. It is not possible for undigested food to turn to body fat, because undigested food does not get absorbed through the intestinal wall. The only effect undigested food can have on your body is to change the consistency of your stools.

Furthermore, as we've seen time and again, enzymes are proteins; fruit enzymes are no exception. **All dietary proteins are treated the same way—shredded beyond recognition and absorbed in tiny parts.**

There is no way "fruit enzymes" could have any activity on undigested food, because they would have been destroyed first.

The Banana-Milk Diet. If nothing else, this diet has simplicity going for it. It allows you 1000 calories per day, in the form of six bananas and three glasses of milk. The diet is generally low in vitamins and minerals, and particularly miserly with regard to iron and protein. It also clearly fails to provide any long-term lifestyle for general health and weight maintenance.

The Fit For Life Diet. The basis for the Fit For Life diet is the assumption that the body's digestive system works in shifts, three eight-hour shifts to a day. These shifts, goes the story, reflect cyclical changes your digestive system goes through during the course of a day. The noon-to-8-pm shift is responsible for "appropriation," the 8-pm-to-4-am shift is responsible for "assimilation," and the 4-am-to-noon shift is responsible for "elimination." The upshot of all this is the assertion that your body does best on different types of food during different times of the day; for example, your body does best on only fruit or fruit juice before noon. There is no medical evidence that the body's digestive system works in shifts.

The Journal of Nutritional Education, in a 1986 report, stated that "the dietary recommendations in the book, based on...erroneous statements, are without foundation." The Fit For Life diet is deficient in calcium, zinc, vitamin D, and vitamin B12.

■ **Fad diets are amusing to read about, but can be dangerous for people who follow them. Sometimes the diets themselves are directly harmful. Other times they merely perpetuate misinformation that prevents the believer from developing more scientifically-grounded nutritional habits. Whatever the particular level of harm, fad diets induce people to adopt dietary extremes, and in so doing represent a further step down the road of bad eating.**

EATING DISORDERS

Anorexia and bulimia are complex psychological problems tied to family background, social class, parent-child relationships, sexuality, and a host of other variables and influences. A thorough examination of the psychological side of these disorders—which is essential for a true understanding of them—is beyond the scope of our concern in this book.

We should note, however, that the anorexic or bulimic person suffers from tremendous emotional distress as a result of his or her distorted patterns of thinking and behavior regarding food. People with eating disorders often experience intense feelings of shame, guilt, and depression, and are frequently unable to prevent their conditions from interfering with other aspects of their lives.

Anorexia Nervosa

At the extreme end of the eating-disorder continuum is anorexia nervosa. People are diagnosed as having this condition when they have lost somewhere between fifteen and twenty-five percent of their original body weight, have no physical illnesses to account for the loss, and continue to perceive themselves as fat even as they become more and more emaciated.

Anorexics fall into two roughly equal groups. Those in the first group are called **restrictor** anorexics. They are the ones who maintain their emaciated condition by simply not eating. Those in the second group are called **bulimic anorexics**. They are individuals who, while falling within the diagnostic criteria for anorexia outlined above, also have episodes arising out of the disorder known as bulimia.

Bulimia

Bulimics engage in what is commonly called the **binge and purge** cycle. Although obsessively concerned with weight, the bulimic regularly loses control and eats very large quantities of food in a short period of time, then uses one or more methods to make up for having binged. These methods include self-induced vomiting **(purging)**, laxatives, diuretics, amphetamines, and excessive exercise. The major difference between bulimic anorexics and simple bulimics is *body weight*—bulimics stay within roughly ten percent of normal body weight (either above or below), while bulimic anorexics take their weight down into the anorexic range described above.

Eating disorders vary in intensity, and some people engage in only certain aspects of the disordered behavior patterns. For example, one group of individuals engages in bulimic purging be-havior, but does not share the bulimic's obsessive fear of weight gain. These are people who purge for specific and comprehensible reasons—for example, a jockey who has to weigh in before the race, or an actress who has a photo session the next morning. Another group loses control and binges, but does not get into purging or any of the other compensatory behaviors.

The actual prevalence of eating disorders in the general population is unknown. Anorexics can be identified by their appearance, but bulimics look "normal" and generally keep their bulimic behavior a secret. At least ninety percent of anorexics are female, and most of these are between fourteen and eighteen years old. They are also most often, but by no means always, white and middle class.

Bulimic behavior is similarly more common among females than males, though by a smaller margin—although again, the actual figures are unknown. Finally, research indicates that the incidence of bulimic behavior is significantly higher among female athletes than female non-athletes. Coaches and others closely connected to female athletes should be aware of this potential problem, and be sensitive to indications that it might be taking place.

The Physical Consequences of Eating Disorders

Up to fifteen percent of anorexics die from the disease. Although the death rate among bulimics is unknown (again, because the incidence of the "secret" disorder itself is unknown), people do die from bulimia, even without losing enough weight to qualify as anorexics. The reason: cardiac arrest.

Short of death, the severity of the physical consequences depends on how abnormal the overeating and purging patterns have become. Even *without* any purging behavior, repeated binge eating alternated with periods of starvation may impair the body's ability to maintain homeostasis by giving the body mixed signals and not allowing it to control intake and output.

When binging is regularly followed by vomiting, the two come to be experienced as one behavior. Satiety, or fullness, no longer works as a signal to stop eating. Larger and larger amounts of food become necessary to eliminate the feeling of hunger. And even small meals begin to *feel* incomplete until they are vomited.

Prolonged vomiting, laxative abuse or diuretic abuse can have many serious physical consequences. Each of these practices depletes the body's supply of chemicals and fluids (including the vital **electrolytes**, especially potassium) needed for the proper functioning of the heart, muscles, and internal organs.

The results can include swollen salivary glands, dryness of the mouth, throat irritation, muscle spasms, muscle fatigue, dizziness, confusion, cardiac irregularities, seizures, and even death.

Laxatives and diuretics have no permanent effect on weight loss. They cause a loss of fluid rather than fat, and must be continually taken, in increasingly larger quantities, to keep the fluid—and the weight—from coming back.

Diuretics, however, cause loss of certain minerals in the urine, especially potassium, which can lead to irregular heart rhythms and death. Laxatives can induce a condition similar to spastic colitis, in which the bowel no longer functions efficiently.

Prolonged vomiting can cause damage and bleeding in the esophagus. It can also cause tooth decay, as a result of the strong stomach acids coming in contact with the teeth.

Other possible consequences of anorexia and bulimia include anemia, vitamin and mineral deficiencies, impaired kidney function, and amenorrhea (cessation of the menstrual cycle).

Getting Help for Eating Disorders

Eating disorders are serious business—they can seriously damage both mind and body. Athletes, who usually pay closer attention to their bodies than do non-athletes, may also be at greater risk for developing eating disorders. **The long-term costs of these behaviors are high; the benefits to athletic performance are few.** Anyone—athlete or not—who has some level of eating disorder should seek professional help at the earliest possible moment.

Help is available from clinics and support groups located in most parts of the country.

- **If you or someone you know has an eating disorder, call your doctor, your local hospital, or your local office of the American Medical Association, and tell them you need help. They will be able to tell you where to find it.**

DANGEROUS NUTRITIONAL PRACTICES

When you think about it, it's amazing how resilient your body is. You can abuse it in all sorts of ways (at least for a while)—by eating badly, getting too little sleep, drinking too much alcohol, smoking, getting sunburned, not exercising—and it will still bounce back.

Push your body too far, though, and the consequences may be dire.

For example, the **Fad Diets** section pointed out that while none of the diets delivered what they promised, they varied in their potential for damaging the dieter's health. Some of the diets were ineffective but harmless; others—the ones calling for more extreme practices—were capable of causing serious physical problems and even death.

What is true for fad diets is true for nutritional practices in general. Some practices, while ineffective, are harmless. For instance, although the athlete who consumes bee pollen probably receives no actual physical benefit, he or she certainly suffers no harm. That is because bee pollen contains nothing to seriously disrupt the body's balances.

Some other practices, however, are not so benign. These practices can throw the body seriously out of balance in a number of ways, with very harmful results.

Fasting

Fasting is not always a bad thing to do, nor is it always dangerous. However, fasting—even short-term fasting—*can* be dangerous for some people, and long- term fasting *can* be dangerous for many people. Fasting involves enough significant risks that it should only be undertaken in consultation with a doctor.

There are many variations the practice.

It can mean eating nothing at all, or only eating a little. It can mean drinking only water, or it can mean subsisting on juices. A fast can be as short as one day or as long as forty days or more. The effects on the body, as well as the potential risks, vary along with the different practices.

What Fasting is Supposed to Do

A great many claims, both reasonable and unreasonable, are made for the benefits of fasting. The only reasonable claim for fasting is that it helps you lose weight. Less reasonable claims for fasting include:

■ *It will help you lose lots of weight quickly and keep it off.* It will cause you to lose weight quickly, all right, but you'll put it right back on when you start eating again.

■ *It gives your digestive system a rest.* This is true but so what? There is no evidence that a "rested" digestive system functions any better (or indeed functions any differently) from an "unrested" digestive system.

   This is like saying you should periodically empty out your gas tank to give the tank a "rest" from holding gasoline. Your gas tank is *made* to hold gasoline, and giving it a rest does not improve its functioning. Similarly, your digestive system is *made* to handle food, and giving it a rest does not improve its functioning, either.

■ *It helps your body "clean out" accumulated "toxins."* This is an emotional-sounding but meaningless phrase.

■ *It will slow the aging process.* Chronically underfed laboratory rats seem to live longer than adequately fed rats. No one knows why. This may have given rise to the *fasting slows the aging process* idea. Does the fact that underfed rats seem to live longer mean that fasting slows the aging process? No one knows.

Extended fasting is sometimes used in the medically supervised treatment of massive obesity. Doctors feel the risks of long-term fasting (which we'll examine in a moment) are outweighed by the risks of continued obesity—in particular, the risk of heart failure.

Side Effects

Fasting *can* be harmful. It is dangerous for people with diabetes, kidney disease or heart disease. Also, pregnant women shouldn't fast, because they must continually supply nutrients to the fetus. For similar reasons, lactating women shouldn't fast, either.

Possible side effects of fasting are fatigue, depression, nausea, hair loss, drying of the skin, muscle cramps, bad breath, liver problems, and diminished interest in sex. Extended fasting (in excess of forty days) has produced electrolyte disorders, protein deficiency, anemia, and malabsorption of Vitamin B12. Some researchers also believe that, under certain circumstances, fasting may increase the risk of stomach cancer.

The truth about fasting is that some people derive some benefits (probably psychological) from doing it for a day, or a few days, at a time. Done in moderation, fasting is not harmful to people who have verified with their doctors that it will not aggravate any existing medical condition.

Fasting is not a desirable way to lose weight, however, because:

- the large initial loss will be of water, which will come back when the person resumes eating

- weight loss, if it is going to be permanent, should not exceed about two pounds per week

- it does not promote life-long habits of good eating

Keep in mind, also, that prolonged fasting can affect the body like anorexia. Starvation is starvation—the body does not know its occupant's reasons for not eating. Although the fasting person is presumably not acting out of a distorted psychological perception of his or her body, and is thus more able to resume normal eating at the appropriate time, the serious fasting enthusiast may lose objectivity and run the risk of harmful effects. This is another reason, especially with regard to extended fasting, to act under medical supervision.

- **Some people derive some benefits (probably psychological) from fasting for a day, or a few days, at a time.**

- **Done in moderation, fasting is not harmful to people *who have verified with their doctors that it will not aggravate any existing medical condition.* Prolonged fasting carries with it serious health risks.**

- **Most of the more exotic claims for fasting—such as *prolonging life*—are unsupported.**

■ **Fasting is not a desirable way to lose weight, because:**

❑ **the large initial loss will be of water, which will come back when you resume eating**

❑ **it triggers the *starvation response* in your body, which may increase your tendency to store fat after you resume eating**

❑ **it promotes lean tissue (muscle) loss as well as fat loss**

Becoming Dehydrated

Because lean body tissue contains a higher proportion of water than does fat tissue, the body of a well-conditioned athlete may contain more water than that of a non-athlete. In fact, the athlete may carry seventy percent or more of his or her weight as water, compared to fifty-five to sixty percent for the average non-athlete.

Water plays a crucial role in athletic performance, discussed in detail in Chapter 14. For the moment, let's just consider the basics of how dehydration occurs and the physical problems it causes.

When you begin to exercise, you begin losing water through sweating and increased breathing. The body decreases the production of urine during prolonged exercise, conserving some water, but the amount of water in the body decreases nonetheless. And since the salt content of sweat is *always* less than the salt content of plasma, water losses from sweat and from the lungs always *increase* the salt concentration in your body.

Dehydration occurs mostly because people drink in response to being thirsty, and thirst is a very inaccurate indicator of the body's need for water.

After a day of exercise, you may take up to three days to rehydrate completely if you drink on the basis of thirst alone. This state of incomplete rehydration is called **involuntary hypohydration**, and the effect can be cumulative: if you fail to rehydrate adequately after a day of exercising you can become even *more* dehydrated after exercising the next day, and still more dehydrated the following day, and so on.

Heat Stroke

One of the most serious dangers of dehydration is **heat stroke**. Heat stroke happens when the normal controls on body temperature no longer work, and body temperature rises to a level which inhibits the regular functioning of the body's cells.

Here's how it works:

During exercise, your body generates heat, and must dissipate that heat to stay at normal body temperature. It does this primarily by sweating, using evaporation to cool you off.

A number of things can interfere with this cooling process, however. For example, if the climate is extremely humid, your sweat will not evaporate and the cooling effect will be lost. Similarly, wearing too much clothing can interfere with evaporation and inhibit the cooling process.

When an athlete becomes dehydrated during exercise, several compensatory mechanisms kick in. First, the production of urine goes way down in an effort to conserve water. Then, because dehydration causes an excess of salt in the fluids around the cells, water from *inside* the cells moves outside the cells in an attempt to equalize the salt balance between the cells and their surroundings. This exodus of cellular fluid causes a degree of dehydration within the cells themselves.

When this cellular dehydration becomes bad enough, it impairs the functioning of these cells, and the athlete experiences impaired performance. In some people at this point, for reasons not understood, the sweating mechanism abruptly *shuts off*.

If the sweating mechanism is shut off, the primary method for heat dissipation is gone. No evaporation takes place, the body temperature rises quickly—often to 108 degrees or even higher. When that happens, the consequences are severe brain damage, kidney failure, heart failure, and death. Every year a few athletes die this way, most commonly during pre-season football training.

As dangerous as dehydration is, it is easily avoidable through careful attention to climate, clothing, and water intake. The program for **Nutrition During Athletic Competition**, in Chapter

20, will help you avoid the problems resulting from dehydration and the extreme imbalances it brings about.

■ **Becoming dehydrated can severely impair athletic performance. In extreme cases, it can be life-threatening.**

■ **Thirst is *not* a good indicator of the need for water. Relying on thirst alone can lead to inadequate rehydration after exercise.**

■ **Guideline for optimum athletic nutrition:**

❑ **Maintain an adequate fluid intake during and after exercise, as detailed in Chapter 20. Ignore any recommendations that restricting water intake will improve performance. These are patently false and can lead to possibly life-threatening dehydration.**

Bodybuilders' Pre-Contest Practices

Often, it is a *combination* of practices, undertaken over a period of months, that pose danger to their practitioners. The practitioners in this case are serious competitive bodybuilders.

If you read bodybuilding magazines, you will get the impression that bodybuilders are all into good nutrition, and are very careful about what they eat. Surprisingly (and unfortunately), this is true only for a minority of bodybuilders.

Most watch their diets only during the two or three months preceding their next contest. When no contest is coming up, they eat whatever they want, and usually put on a lot of fat even though they continue to build muscle by working out. It is common for bodybuilders to be as much as thirty or forty pounds overweight by the time they start dieting for a contest.

The typical competitive bodybuilder follows a program something like this:*

Dieting

Ten or twelve weeks prior to the contest, he starts watching his calories. He enters this period carrying perhaps thirty extra pounds of fat from poor eating habits during his "off season."

If he's really disciplined, he weighs his food before eating it, and keeps a log of everything he eats. He starts by cutting down to about 1000 calories a day, then decreasing from there.

By three to four weeks before the contest, he's eating very little—perhaps one or two small pieces of baked skinless chicken, and maybe a little bit of potato—during the entire day. He may or may not be taking vitamin and mineral supplements. He is probably taking protein supplements in the mistaken belief that by getting lots of dietary protein he will "spare" the protein in his muscles. (Refer back to Chapter 4 if you need a refresher on why this doesn't work.) As he restricts calories this way, he continues to work out very hard.

During this "dieting" period, he may take anabolic steroids to keep his muscles big. He believes the steroids will make his body burn up proportionately more fat and less muscle as it makes up for the deficit of calories. He may also take thyroid pills or shots to speed up the weight loss, and cocaine or some kind of *speed* to work out harder.

As this period goes on, he gets more and more irritable. He may feel as if his brain is not working correctly—his moods swing wildly, until finally he just feels mean and nasty from not eating enough. It's a very trying period psychologically.

Depletion

A week to ten days before the show, he cuts his calories down to almost nothing, but continues to work out hard—many hours on the stationary bicycle, three 90-minute workouts in the gym each day. All of this is geared toward reducing bodyfat as much as possible. During this period he feels very bad, sometimes even sick.

---

*Female bodybuilders generally employ a similar but less severe version of these practices. Since the intent of this section is only to illustrate the kinds of practices bodybuilders use, and not to point out the relatively minor differences between male and female versions, we detail only the male version here.

Three to five days before the contest, he enters the most critical phase. He does three things at once: eats a lot of carbohydrates, eliminates sodium, and severely restricts his intake of water.

His goal is to get as much water out of his body as possible, so water in the skin will not "smooth him out," and he can have maximum definition at contest time. He also stops working out during this period, and lets his body rest up for the contest.

Carbohydrate Loading

On this day he can start eating his normal mix of foods again, but dares not eat a lot—too much would interfere with flexing his abdominal muscles.

Fifteen minutes or so before going onstage, he works out backstage with weights. This gives him a tighter and more intense pump than a normal workout. He may also drink a little bit of wine, if the contest rules allow, to increase his look of vascularity.

When the contest is over, he eats enormous amounts of food, partly out of hunger and partly out of a feeling of deprivation over the preceding two to three months. He keeps working out, but with no contest coming up, again lets himself put on extra fat. By the time the next contest approaches, he is again thirty pounds overweight, and has to repeat the whole cycle.

Contest Day

What are the dangers in this months-long pattern of behavior?

The first danger is the **excess bodyfat**. Every time you go on roller-coaster weight changes, you increase your percentage of bodyfat. For example, if you go from 210 pounds to 180 then back to 210 again, the second time you are at 210 you will have a *higher percentage of bodyfat* **than you did the first time you were at 210.**

The second danger is the **severe reduction of calories**. The reduction is often so pronounced it almost constitutes fasting, and all the dangers that go with fasting come into play.

If a bodybuilder already has diabetes, kidney disease, or heart disease, this kind of dieting can be very dangerous. Even without such a pre-existing condition, the bodybuilder who eats next to nothing for weeks at a time runs the risk of nutritional deficiencies, electrolyte imbalance, anemia, and protein deficiency.

The Dangers

In addition, certain physical affects—such as nausea, fatigue and muscle cramps—as well as certain psychological effects—such as depression—may interfere with a bodybuilder's ability to workout at competitive intensity.

The third danger is **dehydration**. As discussed earlier in this chapter, dehydration can impair the normal activity of certain cells. This danger may be offset to some extent by the fact that the water restriction is begun at the same time workouts are stopped. However, any pronounced dehydration—even in the absence of exercise—can be damaging to the body.

The final danger is the most obvious—**drug use**. Drug use among athletes is a complicated and vitally important subject, which deserves more careful attention than a few sentences in this section could provide. So, rather than get into that discussion here, we direct your attention to Chapter 12, dedicated solely to the subject of drug use among athletes.

■ **The regimen typically followed by bodybuilders before a contest contains a number of health-threatening practices, many of which do not accomplish what they are intended to. Primary dangers include:**

❑ **risk of nutritional deficiencies, electrolyte imbalance, anemia, and protein deficiency as a result of** *severe caloric restriction*

❑ *increased fat storage* **as a result of the extreme oscillations in body weight**

❑ *dehydration* **as a result of restricted water intake**

❑ **decreased training intensity, as a secondary effect of all of the above**

❑ **drug side-effects**

■ Guideline for optimum athletic nutrition:

❑ Follow the Pre-Contest
Bodybuilding Nutritional Program
detailed in Chapter 22. It will get
you massive and ripped without
subjecting you to the dangers—and
failings—of the typical
bodybuilding nutritional regimen.

❖   ❖   ❖

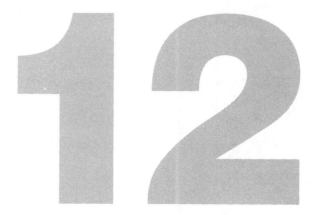

ATHLETES AND DRUGS

As a serious athlete, you will undoubtedly be exposed to drugs at some point, and perhaps will be tempted to give them a try. So, our survey of bad nutrition concludes with a look at drug use among athletes. The purpose of this chapter is not to moralize, but to discuss what drugs athletes take, why they take them, and what the drugs' effects are.

It is easy to understand why drug use among athletes is so common. Athletes—especially serious competitive athletes—operate under intense pressure. Because the smallest advantage can make the difference between winning and losing, athletes frequently believe they have no choice but to take drugs if they are to remain competitive.

Unfortunately, this perception is sometimes correct. The defensive lineman playing under an amphetamine-induced "rage" may indeed be more effective than his drug-free counterpart. The bodybuilder using anabolic steroids may in fact be able to build bigger muscles than would be possible without the drugs.

The question in such instances is not whether drugs give the athlete the competitive edge—it is whether having the competitive edge is worth taking the drugs.

If athletic competition is something to be encouraged, then athletes should not be put in the position of having to choose between using and losing. The only answer is to eliminate drug use altogether, so no one gains an unfair advantage. That is the purpose of drug testing, which is becoming more and more sophisticated and widely used.

It is doubtful, however, that testing will soon catch up with athletes' ingenuity and determination to excel at any cost. So for now, it is important that athletes have reliable information about the difficult choices they face.

ATHLETIC DRUG USE: AN HISTORICAL PERSPECTIVE

Although the controversy over drug use in sports has grown dramatically in recent years, the practice is not new. Athletes as far back as ancient Greece, Rome, and Egypt used various potions and substances to enhance performance. For over 2,000 years, athletes have attempted to augment their physical capabilities by following special diets or ingesting particular substances.

Only relatively recently, however, as chemical technology has become more sophisticated, has drug use become widespread. In the late 1800's, competitive cyclists were the best-known drug users. The grueling six-day bicycle races of that period placed extreme physical and psychological demands on these athletes, and many turned to stimulants of one sort or another for support.

Caffeine, cocaine, heroin, and even strychnine were among the substances frequently used. The same substances were often taken by boxers in this period.

In the early years of the twentieth century, money and gambling began to play bigger roles in boxing and other sports. As the financial stakes grew larger, so did the incentive to boost performance with drugs. Since many drugs were available over the counter, and no testing was done, the use of drugs—especially among professional athletes—continued uncontrolled throughout the early part of the century.

Amphetamine-like stimulants, introduced in the 1930's, offered athletes a new world of performance enhancement. These stimulants were developed extensively during World War II, and were given to the troops to keep them alert and delay fatigue. After the war, stimulant use in sports dramatically increased as the soldiers came home and the prize money continued to grow.

It was not until the 1960's however, that the current controversy over drug use really began.

At the 1960 Olympics, twenty-three year old Danish cyclist Knud Jensen died during time trials after taking amphetamines. In 1967, Tommy Simpson, a twenty-nine year old world-class cyclist, died during the Tour de France, also after taking amphetamines. In 1968, the International Olympic Committee began random drug testing at the Olympic games in Grenoble and Mexico City.

Over the next ten years, many athletes were disqualified from important competitions because of positive tests for amphetamines. Eight weightlifters were disqualified from the 1970 World Weightlifting Championships; seven athletes were disqualified from the 1972 Munich Olympic Games; a distance runner was disqualified from the 1975 Pan-American Games; a cross-country skier lost a bronze medal at the 1976 Innsbruck Olympic Games.

Many officials believed the program of random drug testing was bringing the problem under control, but they were wrong. What was actually happening was that athletes were simply switching to drugs which were either not yet on the banned list or not yet detectable by testing. Most prevalent among those alternative drugs during this period were anabolic steroids.

Although the International Amateur Athletics Federation and the U.S. Amateur Athletic Union banned anabolic steroids in 1970 and 1971 respectively, it was not until 1974 that the **radioimmunoassay** method of steroid testing was shown to be effective.

The International Olympic Committee quickly added anabolic steroids to their rapidly increasing list of banned drugs, and eight athletes—seven of whom were weightlifters—were disqualified for steroid use at the 1976 Olympic games in Montreal. In the following years, a large number of athletes from many different countries were disqualified from competitions on the basis of steroid use.

In the last few years, cocaine has surfaced as a prevalent drug among athletes. A number of major league baseball players have sought treatment for cocaine abuse. The most tragic case was that of college basketball star Len Bias, who died from cocaine use within hours of being drafted by the Boston Celtics.

All of these events have contributed to the present widespread public concern about drug use by athletes. With this background in mind, let's take a look at the various drugs and see:

■ whether they do or do not enhance performance

- what side effects they might have
- what the long-term effects of their use might be

STIMULANTS

Athletes generally use stimulants in hopes of increasing alertness, prolonging exercise endurance, and delaying the onset of fatigue. Stimulants have been most popular in sports where aerobic endurance is critical, such as cycling and soccer. Additionally, some stimulants produce a "rage" response, which has made them popular among athletes in sports such as football, where increased aggression is an asset.

Not all stimulants are alike, of course, and their status in law and sport varies considerably. Some—such as amphetamines—are illegal in most countries. Others—such as caffeine—are legal and freely available. To understand the basic differences among stimulants, let's consider the ways the various drugs achieve their physiological and psychological effects.

Sympathomimetic Amines

Your body reacts to stress through its **sympathetic nervous system**—the system responsible for the **fight-or-flight** response. That system, in response to stress, releases several hormones (*adrenalin, noradrenaline,* and *corticosteroids*) which, together, result in increased heart output, more blood to your muscles, and higher blood sugar levels. These effects ensure that your muscles receive a steady supply of oxygen and nutrients, and that waste products are efficiently removed.

Certain drugs mimic these actions of adrenalin and noradrenaline. Such drugs are called, appropriately enough, **sympathomimetic amines**, because they are *mimetic* of, that is, they mimic, the actions of these compounds released by the sympathetic nervous system.

Many of these can be purchased over the counter. The family of sympathomimetic amines includes *chlorprenaline, ephedrine* (found in *Bronkaid* tablets, *Nyquil,* and several hemorrhoidal preparations), *etafedrine, isoetharine, isoprenaline, methoxyphenamine, methylephedrine,* and similar compounds—all of which have been banned by the International Olympic Committee.

There is little evidence that any of the drugs in this group actually improve athletic performance, and only a few athletes have ever been disqualified for having used them.

Problems in this area usually occur because certain nasal sprays and asthma medications contain sympathomimetic amines as their active ingredients. Athletes using these medications should consult their doctors to avoid unexpected problems, and should be aware that derivatives of the substance *imidazoline*—which does not stimulate the central nervous system—*are* permitted for use as nasal decongestants.

Potential side effects of sympathomimetic amines—at higher than therapeutic doses—include increased blood pressure, nausea, dizziness, and insomnia.

Psychomotor Stimulants

Psychomotor stimulants have roughly the same effect on the sympathetic nervous system as the sympathomimetic amines we just discussed. However, in addition, these drugs affect the *brain*, resulting in a strong feeling of confidence and well-being. As a result, these drugs are very popular among athletes.

Psychomotor stimulants—all of which are banned by the International Olympic Committee—include *amphetamines, benzphetamine, cocaine, dimethylamphetamine, methylamphetamine, norpseudoephedrine, pemoline, phendimetrazine, pipradol, preolintane,* and a large number of other related compounds. Anything thought of as "speed" is almost certainly included in this group.

The psychomotor stimulants influence the athlete's behavior and mood by affecting the activity of **neurotransmitters** in the brain.

Neurotransmitters are chemical compounds that carry messages between the brain cells. Certain neurotransmitters—such as *noradrenaline* and *dopamine*—are linked to behavior and mood. Some psychomotor stimulants, such as *amphetamines*, actually *increase* the production and release of dopamine and noradrenaline, and thereby elevate the athlete's mood. In addition, amphetamines increase the flow of neurotransmitters in the part of the brain that initiates body movement, lowering the threshold for motor activity.

Does all this mean that amphetamines can improve athletic performance?

The answer appears to be *yes, but only to a small degree*. They definitely do not improve athletic *skill*. But, according to the results of some studies, amphetamines appear to prolong *endurance* by perhaps one percent.

That is a very small amount. It can be significant, though, all other things being equal, among athletes at the highest levels of competition. For this reason, this gain is sometimes referred to as the **amphetamine margin.**

The risks to be weighed against this small gain are many and serious—especially when higher doses are taken.

Psychomotor stimulants can affect the cardiovascular system, causing heart palpitations and high blood pressure. They can affect the gastrointestinal system, causing constipation or diarrhea. They can also affect the hormonal system, causing a loss of sex drive and even impotence. During athletic performance, they can mask the physiological signals of overexertion. It was this effect that caused Tommy Simpson to die of heat exhaustion during the 1967 Tour de France.

In addition, psychomotor stimulants are highly addictive. The body quickly develops a tolerance to them, needing larger doses to achieve the same effects. Withdrawal produces severe depression, so the athlete taking them becomes unable to perform without them.

The other disturbing aspect of psychomotor stimulants is that their beneficial effects are not reliable.

These drugs sometimes hinder rather than help athletic performance. Potential negative effects include impaired judgment, insomnia, headaches, and feelings of apathy and depression.

At the extreme negative end of the scale is something called **amphetamine psychosis**—a drug-induced state which closely resembles paranoid schizophrenia. In this condition—which is brought on by large doses of amphetamines—the athlete suffers from hallucinations and feelings of persecution, and may behave irrationally or even aggressively (this is the source of the amphetamine rage referred to above).

Fortunately, the symptoms of amphetamine psychosis go away after drug use is discontinued. However, as with any drug addiction, discontinuing use can be a harrowing and painful experience.

While amphetamine use among athletes appears to have declined in recent years, cocaine use has been on the rise. As the dangers become better understood, and as more well-known athletes continue to acknowledge publicly their inability to control their cocaine use, we may perhaps see a decline in that area also.

Other Central Nervous System Stimulants

The drugs in this category—with the exception of caffeine—are generally quite poisonous and very dangerous to use without close medical supervision.

Included in this group, which is also banned by the International Olympic Committee, are *amiphenazole, bemigride, caffeine, croproamide, crotethamide, doxapram, ethamivan, leptazol, nikethamide, picrotoxin, strychnine, and a number of other related compounds.*

Each of these drugs stimulates some part of the central nervous system, but in high doses can cause convulsions, followed by respiratory failure and death. Because of this risk, most of these drugs have not been widely used by athletes (although two athletes tested positive for nikethamide at the Munich Olympics).

Caffeine

The exception is **caffeine**.

Taken in small doses—such as the amount contained in one or two cups of coffee—caffeine seems to improve alertness and reduce fatigue or drowsiness. It also increases the heart rate, and acts as a diuretic. Injected in large doses, caffeine can induce convulsions.

A great deal of controversy exists over the effect of caffeine on endurance. The theory is that caffeine increases fat oxidation during exercise, thus *sparing* glycogen for use later in the event (this is covered in more detail in *Energy and Endurance*, Chapter 13).

Whether caffeine actually increases endurance is uncertain—studies have yielded mixed results.

Several facts can be stated about caffeine, however:

- A regular user builds up a tolerance to it. The maximum effect is achieved after withdrawal for at least four days.

- Amounts in excess of about 100 to 250 mg. (one or two cups of coffee) increase tension without further increasing alertness or reducing fatigue.

- Caffeine may produce undesirable side effects, including heart palpitations, nervousness, irritability, insomnia, nausea, diarrhea, and headaches.

For a more complete discussion of caffeine, see *Ergogenic Aids*, Chapter 16.

ANABOLIC STEROIDS

For weightlifters and bodybuilders, anabolic steroids are a fact of life. Many, if not most, of these athletes firmly believe it is impossible to win without them. Athletes in other sports—especially those requiring bulk—frequently use anabolic steroids as well.

The Theory Behind Anabolic Steroids

The adult musculature of the human male starts to develop when, at puberty, the testes begin to produce the hormone **testosterone**. Testosterone causes both **anabolic** changes ("building up"; for example, the development of bigger muscles) and **androgenic** changes ("masculinization"; for example, the growth of facial hair and the deepening of the voice).

Additionally, testosterone causes the **epiphyses** (the ends of the growing bones) to seal, preventing the bones from getting longer and halting any further increases in height. Testosterone also brings about changes in primary sexual characteristics, such as the increase in penis size and the initiation of sperm production.

Over the last 50 years, chemists have attempted to devise drugs that imitate the anabolic (building up) effects of testosterone, while minimizing the androgenic (masculinizing) effects. To some extent they have succeeded. Some anabolic steroids have much more muscle-growth effect and much less masculinizing effect than testosterone. However, *all* anabolic steroids have *some* masculinizing effect, and this can cause serious problems.

Clinical Tests vs. Athletes' Experience

An interesting aspect of the steroid question is the wide divergence between scientific findings and athletes' experience. For years, scientific studies have concluded that anabolic steroids do not reliably produce increases in strength or performance. At the same time, bodybuilders know full well that anabolic steroids work. Why this disagreement?

The answer may lie in the way scientists work with human subjects. Human experimentation must be approved in advance by local ethics committees. This means that scientists researching the effects of anabolic steroids must, to get approval for their research, agree to use doses that are proven to be safe. At safe dosage levels, results are indeed unreliable.

However, most athletes taking steroids exceed doses proven to be safe, and are therefore taking doses much larger than can be used in formal experiments. This may account for much of the difference in effect.

Additionally, athletes—especially weightlifters—sometimes use the drugs differently from experimental subjects. Some athletes engage in **stacking** of steroids, in which they use different types of steroids simultaneously. The normal *stacking* pattern is to start with a relatively low dose of one oral anabolic steroid, then increase the dose over a period of weeks while also receiving injections of a second, longer- acting steroid. Some weeks prior to competition, the steroids are dropped in favor of testosterone to avoid detection by testing.

Another theory which may help explain the difference between science and experience is that steroids may in fact not make muscles bigger, but rather extend muscular endurance and recovery ability, allowing harder and longer training periods. More training then brings about bigger muscles.

Even given existing differences of opinion, a significant number of experiments support the belief that anabolic steroids increase muscle *size*. Less settled is whether the increase is due to a buildup of normal muscle tissue or a "bloating" of muscle with water and tissue salts. Some experiments suggest this bloating effect may be the dominant cause of the increase in size.

To the extent anabolic steroids build muscle size through bloating, they do not directly increase muscle strength. However, the psychological aspect must be considered. An athlete who sees himself or herself getting bigger, and *believes* steroids increase muscle strength, may perform better for that reason alone. Several studies have shown that subjects who *thought* they were taking steroids (but who in fact were not) often performed as well as those who actually *were* taking steroids.

Side Effects of Anabolic Steroids

Most athletes who are exposed to anabolic steroids are aware these drugs can cause serious side effects, but many choose to ignore the long-term risks in exchange for immediate gains. It's easy to understand such a decision in the current competitive environment. Regardless, we urge you to consider whether the benefits warrant the risk.

Athletes injecting anabolic steroids sometimes use disposable syringes, but sometimes, instead of throwing the syringes away, they share them with other athletes. **This should NEVER BE DONE, because of the possibility of transmitting the AIDS virus. One case has already been documented of a weight-lifter, who had no history of homosexuality or hard drug abuse, contracting AIDS.**

AIDS

Anabolic steroids can also affect an athlete's general appearance, causing acne, inflamed follicles on the upper back, and a puffy appearance around the face and torso.

Acne

Another danger is that anabolic steroids will contribute to heart disease. They do this two ways:

Heart Disease

■ Steroids reduce the level of high density lipoproteins in the blood (see the discussion of these under *Cholesterol* in Chapter 6), thereby increasing risk of atherosclerosis and in turn the chances of having a heart attack. Recently a twenty-six year old athlete underwent a quadruple bypass necessitated by his severe atherosclerosis from steroid use.

■ Steroids cause salt retention, which can raise blood pressure, increasing the risk of heart failure.

The liver is also subject to damage from anabolic steroid use. The most common problem in this area is **cholestatic jaundice**, a condition in which the skin turns yellow and the liver gradually loses its ability to function. This problem will usually correct itself if steroid use is discontinued in time, but can be fatal.

Liver

Hepatoma (liver cancer) and **peliosis** (pockets of blood in the liver) are less common but even more serious side effects of anabolic steroid use.

Athletes—especially bodybuilders—using steroids also run an increased risk of tendon damage. As bodybuilders suddenly increase the number of pounds their muscles are able to lift, they put additional stress on tendons which were already subject to

Tendon Damage

abnormally high tension. The tendons, having had no time to adapt to the increase, can tear, causing serious disability.

Sexual Functioning

There is no doubt anabolic steroids reduce normal testosterone production. It is unclear, however, whether this reduction can permanently damage normal testicular function. The fear is that without producing its own testosterone, the male reproductive system may simply wither and die. This is not an established side effect, but some scientists believe it is a real danger. Similarly unsettled is whether steroids can result in loss of sexual desire or impotence.

Stunted Growth

A final point concerns the use of anabolic steroids by young athletes. Recall that one of the androgenic effects of steroids is to seal the ends of the bones, preventing further lengthening. This has the effect of stunting the growth of athletes who take steroids before being fully grown.

How young is too young? There's no magic number, but the long leg bones keep growing until about age 20, and certain bones in the chest and back continue to grow for a number of years after that.

Detection of Anabolic Steroid Use

Before 1973, no tests were sensitive enough to detect the very small amounts of steroids present in an athlete's urine. In 1973, however, Professor Raymond Brooks, of St. Thomas' Hospital in London, unveiled the two-stage test still in use today.

Using this test, injectable steroids are detectable for up to several months after being taken. Oral steroids, on the other hand, may be detectable for only a few weeks.

Athletes have responded to the tests in several ways. First, they have kept track of what anabolic agents are detectable, and when possible have simply taken others. Second, they have learned (or believe they have learned) the outer limits of the test's sensitivity, and have been careful to stop using steroids far enough in advance to go undetected. Third, they have started using testosterone to prolong the effects of the steroids they have taken.

Since testosterone occurs naturally in the body, officials have a much harder time determining whether a given level is suspiciously high in a particular individual. However, tests for high levels of testosterone were administered at the 1984 Olympics in Los Angeles.

A recent development is the use of **human chorionic gonadotropin**, or HCG, to boost testosterone production. This substance, present in the urine of pregnant women, boosts testosterone production in men and is likely to be a target of testing in the near future. In the meantime, its advocates claim it boosts performance levels, but the evidence is inconclusive.

HCG

In contrast to sports requiring strength and endurance, some sports, such as target shooting, fencing, and ski-jumping, require calmness and relaxation for maximum performance. To overcome the nervousness that may accompany the pressures of competition, athletes in these and similar sports sometimes turn to drugs for assistance.

ANTI-ANXIETY DRUGS

Some anti-anxiety drugs are currently banned; others are not. Abuse in this area is often difficult to determine, because one person's habit (for example, a glass of wine the evening before a competition) may be another person's rule infraction.

Alcohol is the most frequently used anti-anxiety drug. It is fast acting, and functions as both an anesthetic and a depressant on the central nervous system. In small amounts, it relaxes people and slightly decreases their efficiency. In larger amounts, especially over time, alcohol creates many problems.

Alcohol

Over-consumption of alcohol can cause nausea, dehydration, headache, amnesia, impotence and depression. **It is also toxic to the intestinal tract, and can cause maldigestion and malabsorption of certain nutrients, including folic acid, thiamine, calcium and iron.** Regular drinking also significantly increases the risks of oral cancer and stroke.

Many people don't realize alcohol is addictive. But in fact, the regular drinker develops a tolerance to alcohol, as well as a physical and psychological dependency. Quitting alcohol can be as hard as quitting many other addictive drugs.

Even in moderation, alcohol tends to impair judgment, reduce motor coordination and slow reaction times. Hangovers interfere with vision, concentration and stamina. Accordingly, alcohol use may be counterproductive for many sports.

Minor Tranquilizers

Some athletes have turned to tranquilizers as a means of reducing anxiety. These drugs appear to accomplish that goal without impairing judgment and coordination.

A drug, *meprobamate*, and a family of drugs, the *benzodiazepines*, are held in particular favor. Meprobamate blocks particular nerve pathways in the brain, and reduces anxiety without producing drowsiness. However, meprobamate is addictive, and reduces tolerance to alcohol.

The benzodiazepines (*Valium, Librium*) are *sedatives*, originally developed for reducing aggression in tigers (believe it or not) so they could be tamed. Although these drugs generally do not present dangers of toxicity or harmful side effects, they are habit-forming, and can be very difficult to stop taking. Withdrawal symptoms can include depression, nightmares and hallucinations.

The International Olympic Committee has not yet banned these drugs, in spite of their widespread use. This may be because there is no solid evidence that these drugs improve performance.

Beta-Blockers

One of the more creative uses of drugs to steady nerves involves the **beta-blockers**—drugs normally used to treat high blood pressure and certain heart disorders.

The normal physical response to stress includes increased heart rate, triggered by release of adrenalin. Adrenaline binds to what are known as the **beta receptors**, specific sites on the heart that help control heart rate. As a result of this binding, the heart speeds up.

The beta-blockers are drugs that interfere with the action of adrenaline on the beta receptors. In the presence of beta-blockers, adrenaline doesn't cause the heart to speed up. The beta-blockers include *propranolol*, *practolol*, and *sotalol*.

Many sharpshooters and archers take beta-blockers to improve their aims. By slowing their heart rate, they have more time to fire *between* beats. Firing between beats allows the sharpshooter to fire without the minute jiggle produced by the heart beat. This, it is claimed, significantly increases accuracy.

Another use, as mentioned above, is to improve relaxation. Many giant slope ski jumpers have taken *propranolol* for this reason. One of the foreseeable problems of slowing down your heart beat is that you may no longer supply enough blood to the brain and may faint. The *Agony of Defeat* ski jumper in the opening segments of *ABC's Wide World of Sports* is said to have taken a beta-blocker, and fainted just as he started down the slope. Needless to say, in this instance it did not improve his performance (although it *did* result in some spectacular footage).

Beta-blockers affect other parts of the body, however, and the full extent of their effects is unknown.

Potential side effects of beta-blockers include heart failure, depression, weakness, fatigue, nausea, and impotence. These potentially harmful effects make beta-blockers very risky to use if not under medical supervision.

Nicotine

Many people, whether athletes or not, smoke tobacco to relax. They find the nicotine in tobacco smoke produces a calming effect. However, most athletes are aware of the hazards of smoking—bronchitis, lung cancer, and heart disease, to name a few—and feel smoking will hurt their performance overall more than help it.

Surprisingly enough, in light of all the research on smoking, there are few scientific studies closely analyzing the effects of smoking on athletic performance. Perhaps this is one area in which knowledge of the dangers is so widespread that athletes simply don't need to be convinced that smoking is not in their competitive interest.

Marijuana

Although many people smoke marijuana to relax, little research has been done on marijuana's effects on athletic performance. The drug's known physiological effects point in both directions—some suggest performance might be improved; others suggest it would be hindered.

Because marijuana both induces **tachycardia** (fast heart beat) and releases carbon monoxide into the blood, it is thought that smoking marijuana reduces capacity for work. The small amount of research done in this area seems to support this conclusion.

At the same time, other effects of marijuana smoking include bronchodilatation (opening up of air passages in the lungs), increased blood flow to exercising muscles, and possibly decreased perception of fatigue. While these factors suggest marijuana might increase the athlete's capacity for work, as yet no research has found this to be the case.

Painkillers

In today's highly competitive atmosphere, athletes begin training younger, and continue training longer and harder, than ever before. As the same body parts go through the same motions over and over, inevitably the gradual wear takes its toll. Overuse injuries—especially to tendons, ligaments, and joints—are increasingly common.

Many athletes are unwilling to stop and rest when their bodies are in pain, and so turn to painkillers to allow them to continue training or competing. This can be very dangerous, since pain is the body's way of telling the athlete that something is wrong. "Playing with pain" may be admirable in terms of the athlete's determination, but sometimes foolish in terms of the athlete's true best interests.

Local Anesthetics

One of the more dangerous practices is use of long-lasting local anesthetics prior to a competition or an extended workout. These drugs—such as *procaine* (trade name *Novocain*), *lidocaine* (trade name *Xylocaine*), and *bupivacaine* (trade name *Marcaine*)—"deaden" the affected area for a number of hours after being injected.

This practice presents two main risks:

- The athlete may worsen an existing injury, or sustain additional injuries, without knowing it. The loss in either case may be much more costly than the loss from resting would have been.

- **Local anesthetics can cause abnormal heart rhythms**, and larger doses can cause convulsions and even death.

Anti-Inflammatory Drugs

Any athlete who has suffered an injury is familiar with the swelling, redness, and pain that accompanies damage to tissue. This group of symptoms is known as the **inflammatory response,** and is caused by the release of certain chemicals called **prostaglandins.**

Anti-inflammatory drugs block the synthesis of prostaglandins, and so prevent the inflammatory response. The best known of these drugs is *aspirin*, or acetylsalicylic acid. Aspirin is inexpensive, it's safe, and it works very well. It can cause gastrointestinal problems, but only if taken in high doses over substantial periods of time.

Another group of anti-inflammatory drugs, reportedly used by many football and basketball players, is not so benign.

These drugs—including *indomethacin, oxyphenbutazone*, and *phenylbutazone* (sometimes referred to as "bute") are stronger than aspirin, but can cause serious side effects. Diarrhea is one common response. Continued use can cause ulcers in the stomach or intestines, as well as headaches, dizziness and confusion.

Indomethacin, oxyphenbutazone, and *phenylbutazone* have become quite controversial in the last few years following consumer groups' claims that the drugs have caused thousands of deaths worldwide. The British government has already responded by imposing tighter restrictions on the use of oxyphenbutazone. In the U.S., the Food and Drug Administration is looking into the matter, and is likely to issue similar restrictions in the near future.

Corticosteroids

Corticosteroids are natural substances produced by the adrenal glands in response to stress. They reduce inflammation, and so are also taken as drugs for the treatment of arthritis and other inflammatory diseases. Athletes use corticosteroids by injecting them directly into an injured area, to reduce pain and swelling.

There are two basic categories of corticosteroids:

■ **glucocorticoids**—such as *cortisol, hydrocortisone*, and *corticosterone*—which help suppress the inflammatory response, and also facilitate more efficient formation of glucose from protein

■ **mineralocorticoids**—such as aldosterone—which help control the body's balance of salt and water by affecting kidney function

Corticosteroids can operate as both painkillers and stimulants. In addition to reducing inflammation, these drugs sometimes create feelings of well-being or euphoria. However, as is so often the case, corticosteroids have a serious down side.

Side Effects

Continued use of corticosteroids can cause the same kinds of psychotic reactions associated with other stimulants, as well as a host of physical problems. Among the physical problems are accumulation of body fat in characteristic locations ("moon face," "buffalo hump"), muscle weakness (which may be permanent), insomnia, cataracts, osteoporosis, and higher susceptibility to infection.

Regular corticosteroid users may also face serious difficulties in discontinuing use of the drugs.

This is not because corticosteroids are addicting—they aren't—but rather because regular use of corticosteroids can inhibit the pituitary gland's production of **ACTH** (adrenocorticotropic hormone), which controls the *natural* production of corticosteroids in the adrenal cortex.

With ACTH production inhibited, the adrenal cortex may no longer function properly. The athlete who abruptly ceases taking corticosteroids may suffer from **adrenal insufficiency**—which can cause weakness, confusion, low blood pressure, dehydration, nausea, vomiting, and diarrhea. Accordingly, athletes may have to gradually decrease corticosteroid use rather than stop it all at once.

A related practice adopted by some athletes is taking ACTH itself, rather than corticosteroids, to stimulate the *natural* production of corticosteroids in the adrenal cortex. This practice has caused serious illnesses, most notably among racing cyclists.

Narcotic Analgesics

In contrast to local anesthetics and anti-inflammatory drugs, both of which act primarily on the injured area, the narcotic analgesics act on the cerebral cortex of the brain to eliminate pain *generally*. Included in this group are the "hard drugs"—*morphine, heroin, methadone,* and a host of derivative and related synthetic compounds. In addition to being banned from athletic competition, of course, these drugs are almost universally illegal.

Morphine—the active ingredient in opium—quashes pain and anxiety while creating feelings of euphoria. It produces an initial stimulant effect, followed by a reduction in physical coordination and a sedative effect. Morphine is highly addictive, tolerance develops quickly, and withdrawal is very uncomfortable. *Heroin*, a derivative of morphine, is considerably more powerful.

Although the dangers of these narcotic drugs are well known, the drugs have sometimes been used by athletes—especially boxers and cyclists—for their anesthetic and stimulant effects. Fortunately, this practice does not appear to be common today.

A more difficult question is whether *codeine* should be prohibited for use by athletes. *Codeine*, like morphine, is an opiate, but is clearly much less dangerous. It is considerably weaker, has fewer side effects, is not as addictive, and is routinely prescribed by doctors as a general analgesic (painkiller). It can even be purchased over the counter in some countries. However, because it is an opiate, codeine is still banned by the International Olympic Committee.

The brain produces its own form of morphine: **endorphins**. Endorphins are natural substances which, when released, bind to certain receptor sites in the central nervous system (not unlike the way adrenalin binds to beta-receptors in the tissues of the heart in response to stress) and block the sensations of pain. It appears morphine may bind to the very same receptor sites; thus, opiates may work by imitating a natural process in the body.

Runner's high is probably caused by a release of endorphins. This can have its drawbacks, however, as the endorphins can mask pain and discomfort during running, allowing a runner to run longer than advisable and increasing potential for injury.

DRUGS AND FEMALE ATHLETES

Performances by female athletes have improved dramatically in recent decades. As women have been afforded the opportunity to train more seriously, they have set new records in almost all sports at a pace much faster than that of men.

Women's top performances today already equal those of men in recent decades, and the gap is closing. Although women may never be able to perform at the same level as men in sports based on pure physical strength, it is very likely female athletes will eventually compete in many areas on equal terms with men.

All of these developments are positive, but they also mean women athletes are now more than ever subject to the same competitive pressures as men. As a result, most of the drug-related concerns discussed in this chapter apply to female athletes just as much to males. In addition, women have certain concerns that are theirs exclusively, and those are discussed below.

Women and Anabolic Steroids

Recall from the discussion of anabolic steroids that men naturally produce both anabolic and androgenic steroids after puberty. Women also produce both, but produce androgenic steroids (from their adrenal glands) in such small amounts that they do not bring about the masculinizing effects experienced by men.

So when a man takes anabolic steroids, he simply adds to his existing balance of anabolic and androgenic hormones; when a woman takes anabolic steroids, she *shifts* the balance toward a proportionately higher amount of androgenic hormones. As a result, she may begin to look more like a man.

Several physiologic changes occur.

- Anabolic steroids may supress the female athlete's normal menstrual cycle.
- She may experience **clitoral hypertrophy**—a significant enlargement of the clitoris (paralleling the enlargement of the penis experienced by males during puberty).
- Her vocal cords may lengthen, causing her voice to become deeper.
- She may begin growing hair in ways normally associated only with males (e.g., facial hair).
- She may develop male pattern baldness.

Although the menstrual cycle will normally resume after the drugs are discontinued, the rest of the changes mentioned are usually *irreversible*, and cannot be prevented by taking estrogens (female hormones) while taking anabolic steroids.

Anabolic steroids may also cause birth defects if a woman takes them in high doses during pregnancy. Specifically, they can cause a condition called **pseudohermaphroditism**, in which a female fetus partially develops male sex organs.

Although most female athletes know the dangers of taking drugs during pregnancy, they may take drugs before being aware they are pregnant.

Hormone Manipulation

A related matter is the use of oral contraceptives. For some female athletes, controlling the menstrual cycle may be a way of maximizing performance—many females experience losses in athletic performance immediately before and/or during their periods. By manipulating their hormonal systems in this way, women may gain not only by regulating the physical symptoms associated with menstruation, but also by developing a sense of confidence as a result of being able to control their bodies.

Much speculation has been advanced about how top female gymnasts manage to stay so small for so long. It is not uncommon for female gymnasts in their late teens to have bodies much like those of 11- or 12-year-old girls. Although some drugs, including anabolic steroids, might accomplish this effect, there is no evidence drugs are actually the cause.

The likely explanation is that the gymnasts are manipulating their hormonal systems through diet. In general, girls will not begin menstruating if their bodies are less than about seventeen percent fat. Gymnasts' bodies often contain less than half that amount, because of careful attention to diet. As a result, they remain "girls'" bodies, rather than becoming "women's," much longer than normal.

Gender Testing

Gender testing, while not directly a drug-related issue, is a special concern of female athletes, so we will discuss it here.

As mentioned above, women's athletic performances are getting closer to equaling men's performances in many areas. However, they are not equal yet, and so a man competing in a women's event would, all other things being equal, have an unfair advantage. A number of men—more than one might expect, as a matter of fact—have actually masqueraded as women to exploit that advantage. As a result, sports officials for many years have insisted on verifying that all competitors in female events are actually female.

This verification used to be accomplished by visual inspection. Neither the officials nor the athletes were very happy with that system, however, so more scientific tests were created. Today's tests determine femininity by verifying the presence of **Barr bodies**, chromosomal material that women have but men don't.

These tests are both accurate and respectful of privacy—they can be performed on a sample of skin cells from the athlete's mouth or the root of the athlete's hair.

CURRENT AND FUTURE TRENDS

As drug testing becomes increasingly sophisticated, and more and more drugs become detectable through scientific methods, one might expect drug use among athletes to decrease. However, instead of giving up drugs, athletes have responded to testing by moving to different drugs—those which are as yet undetectable or are not yet banned—and by learning how to tailor their drug use to the sensitivities of the current tests.

This section discusses a few of the current practices among athletes seeking ways to gain that extra edge.

Eleutherococcus

Eleutherococcus is an extract of a plant called *Eleutherococcus senticosus,* which grows wild in the forests of Siberia. Soviet athletes have reportedly been using *Eleutherococcus* as a stamina-building drug for a number of years. Because it does not fall into any of the International Olympic Committee's categories of banned drugs, its use is legal in athletic competition.

Eleutherococcus is reportedly used widely in the Soviet Union by individuals in stressful occupations, or in occupations requiring concentration for extended periods of time. Soviet cosmonauts are reported to have taken the drug during extended stays in space.

It is claimed that *Eleutherococcus* increases endurance, coordination, and concentration, and reduces stress. Western scientists, however, have not been able to verify these claims. A recent Swedish study looked into *Eleutherococcus* and concluded, "It has hitherto been impossible to find documentation confirming that [*Eleutherococcus*] should have a positive effect of athletic performances. The few existing reports on such an effect are not convincing."

Dichloroacetic Acid

Although the research on *dichloroacetic acid* is still in a very early phase, some scientists believe that the substance may enhance endurance by slowing the accumulation of lactic acid in the muscles during exercise (see *Energy and Endurance,* Chapter 13 for an explanation of the role of lactic acid in endurance).

Dichloroacetic acid has produced a pronounced increase in endurance in rats, but neither the benefits nor the side effects for humans is known.

Athletes needing to lose weight to qualify for particular weight categories used to take stimulants, which allowed them to exercise longer while eating less. Since stimulants are now readily detectable through drug testing, athletes have sought other means of quickly shedding unwanted pounds.

Diuretics have been widely used for this purpose. These drugs increase the flow of urine, causing a loss of fluids and, consequently, a loss of weight. Weight remains low until the fluids are replaced. The athlete, therefore, can take the diuretic, weigh in after losing the fluids, then rehydrate by drinking lots of fluids or receiving intravenous infusions.

Although this practice is not banned, it is dangerous. It can cause significant changes in the body's electrolyte balance, which can trigger abnormal heart rhythms.

Another way athletes—especially bodybuilders—attempt to achieve a rapid weight loss is by taking **thyroid drugs.** The thyroid regulates the body's metabolic rate. Thyroid drugs, by stimulating the thyroid, increase the metabolic rate and bring about weight loss by causing fats and carbohydrates to be utilized faster, decreasing the body's reserves of fats and carbohydrates.

As is often the case with drug effects, however, the body follows up by homeostatically compensating in the opposite direction. An athlete who is taking a thyroid drug to promote weight loss, and then stops, may suffer a period of thyroid deficiency during which the metabolic rate will be slower than usual. The athlete will likely regain the lost weight, and may also suffer from other symptoms of hypothyroidism: weakness, fatigue, anemia, cold intolerance, slow heart rate.

Somatotropin, or *growth hormone,* may well replace anabolic steroids as the drug of choice among athletes seeking to increase body size and muscle strength. Its advocates claim somatotropin works better than anabolic steroids, produces longer-lasting gains, and has far fewer side effects.

At the present time there is no reliable method for testing for somatotropin. Once such a method is developed, the drug will most likely be banned from athletic competition.

Somatotropin is also not without risks. Overuse can cause **acromegaly**, a kind of physical deformity characterized by en-

Diuretics

Thyroid Drugs

Human Growth Hormone

largement of the jaws, hands and feet. **In addition, by using a "foreign" growth hormone you may end up producing antibodies to your *own* growth hormone.**

That would mean that your own body's carefully-balanced supply of growth hormone would be destroyed for the rest of your life, and you would become dependent on outside sources of growth hormone—much as a diabetic is dependent on outside sources of insulin.

Finally, recent research indicates that although HGH does increase "muscle size," what's actually increasing is the amount of **connective tissue** surrounding muscle fibers, not the size of the muscle fibers themselves. **The effect of this kind of growth is a decrease in muscle strength**.

Blood Doping

Red blood cell infusion, or **blood doping**, is another example of the ingenious ways in which athletes attempt to improve performance without running afoul of the drug tests.

This method involves two stages:

First, a pint or two of blood is removed from the athlete, and then is frozen and stored. Over the next several weeks, the athlete's bone marrow, stimulated by the loss of the blood, forms more red blood cells and returns the athlete's blood volume to normal.

Then, a day or two before the competition, the stored blood is reinfused into the athlete, creating a *surplus* of red blood cells. With these extra red blood cells, the athlete's blood can carry more oxygen to the muscles. This could theoretically result in more efficient functioning of the muscles and increased endurance.

Research indicates that blood doping actually works. A recent study demonstrated a fifteen percent increase in aerobic performance of middle-distance runners.

However, blood doping is not without its drawbacks. If the blood used is not from the athlete but from a donor, there is the risk of transmission of hepatitis, AIDS, and other blood-borne diseases. Even if the athlete's own blood is used, the risk of infection from the reinfusion procedure is always present. In addition, the increase in red cell number also increases the viscosity (resistance to flow) of the blood, forcing the heart to work harder.

■ **This chapter is in the section on** *Bad Nutrition* **for a reason:**

None of the drugs athletes take to improve athletic performance enhance health and fitness.

The best you can hope for is that the drugs will not seriously injure your health. Since so many of the drugs have negative side effects, and so many of the side effects are quite serious, we hope you will think long and hard before making drugs a part of your program.

❖   ❖   ❖

PART FOUR

NUTRITION AND ATHLETIC PERFORMANCE

This section covers:

—energy production, and how to maximize it;

—the physiological role of water, and the best way to use sports drinks during endurance events to maintain the optimum fluid balance;

—weight control and body composition;

—ergogenic aids.

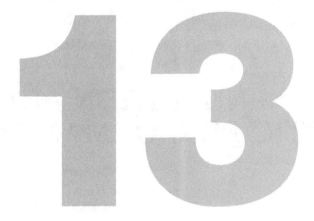

ENERGY AND ENDURANCE

Before skill can produce masterful execution of a spinning roundhouse kick, before strength can contribute to a world-record power lift, there must first be *movement*—and movement requires energy.

Not surprisingly, the basic goal of exercise nutrition is to improve the body's energy production.

This chapter takes a look at the energy production mechanisms in your body. Once you understand how those mechanisms work, you will be in a much better position to evaluate and implement nutritional recommendations.

A note to the technically wary: This chapter is the most complicated in the book. You don't have to read it to use the programs detailed in **Part Five**. If you choose to skip it, do check out the grey summary boxes distributed throughout. They won't give you the full story, but they contain the basic concepts.

ENERGY STORAGE IN THE BODY

Your body uses four different *fuels* for energy production. They differ in the amount of energy they contain and in how quickly they can release their energy. These fuels are:

- ATP
- circulating glucose

- glucose stored as glycogen in the muscles and liver
- fat

(Under certain conditions, protein also serves as energy fuel, but, for reasons we will see later, when possible you want to limit your body's use of it for that purpose.)

ATP stands for **adenosine triphosphate**. ATP *directly* supplies energy for many of the chemical reactions in your body. ATP is fundamentally important—no ATP, no reactions—including muscle contraction.

The *tri* in adenosine *tri*phosphate means each ATP molecule has *three* of something chemists call **phosphates.** (Don't worry about exactly what a phosphate is.) The chemical bonds between these phosphates are known as **high-energy bonds**.

High-energy bonds contain stored energy, in much the same way as a compressed spring contains stored energy. These high-energy bonds can be broken. When broken they *release* their stored energy, just as a compressed spring releases its stored energy when allowed to expand to its normal length. The energy released when a high-energy bond is broken is the energy that powers muscle contraction.

When a high-energy bond is broken, the ATP loses one of its three phosphates, and becomes adenosine *di*phosphate, ADP (*di = two*).

Or, looked at another way,

$$ATP = ADP + a\ phosphate + energy$$

Now, since ATP supplies the energy for all chemical reactions in the body, and since it gets "used up" (turned into ADP) whenever it supplies some of that energy, you need a mechanism for constantly creating new ATP. And that's where the other energy fuels come in. The metabolism of glucose, glycogen, and fat provides the energy for the resynthesis of ATP.

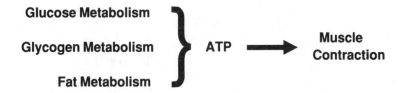

Glucose Metabolism

Glycogen Metabolism   } **ATP** ⟶ **Muscle Contraction**

Fat Metabolism

■ The energy in ATP is stored in its high-energy bonds, and this energy is released when the bonds are broken.

■ ATP directly supplies the energy for muscle contraction, and for many other energy-requiring reactions in the body.

■ Your other *energy fuels*—circulating glucose, glycogen stored in the muscles and liver, and fat—provide the energy for creation of more ATP.

HOW GLUCOSE IS USED TO SYNTHESIZE ATP

Let's see just how glucose is involved in the synthesis of new ATP. Three processes are important here: **glycolysis**, **Krebs Cycle**, and **pyruvate-to-lactate**.

Glycolysis

Glycolysis is the splitting of glucose (*glyco* = glucose, *lysis* = splitting).

When a cell gets the biochemical signal that energy is needed, the glucose goes through a long series of chemical changes in which it is broken down (split) into two molecules, called **pyruvates**.

As the glucose molecule gets broken down, new ATP is created—specifically, for every molecule of glucose broken down, you manufacture two new ATP's.

You can picture glycolysis this way:

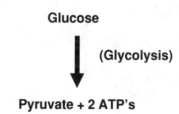

Glucose

(Glycolysis)

Pyruvate + 2 ATP's

> ■ **Three processes contribute to the resynthesis of ATP:** *glycolysis, Krebs Cycle, and pyruvate-to-lactate.*
>
> ■ *Glycolysis* **involves the breakdown of glucose.**
>
> ■ **For every molecule of glucose broken down during glycolysis, you get two new ATP molecules.**

Krebs Cycle

After the glucose has become pyruvate, the pyruvate stands at a fork in the road. It can go one of two ways, and which way it goes is determined by whether there is any **oxygen** available at the moment.

If oxygen *is* available, the pyruvate goes into the second of the three processes—the **Krebs Cycle**. We say the energy production by this mechanism is **aerobic** (*aerobic* literally means "with oxygen").

We need not explore the chemical intricacies of the Krebs Cycle. What's important for our purposes is that for each molecule of glucose that enters the Krebs Cycle, *36 ATP molecules are produced*—a high rate of **energy return** on the glucose invested. Added to the two molecules of ATP produced during glycolysis, that makes a total of 38 ATP's produced by the aerobic energy mechanism.

In addition to ATP, the aerobic process also yields carbon dioxide and water, waste products that are eliminated through the lungs and kidneys.

Putting our first two processes together, we get a picture that looks like this:

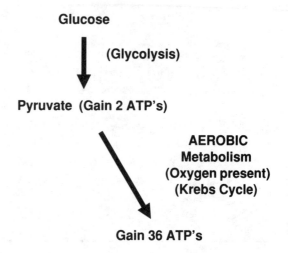

Glucose

(Glycolysis)

Pyruvate (Gain 2 ATP's)

AEROBIC
Metabolism
(Oxygen present)
(Krebs Cycle)

Gain 36 ATP's

■ In the presence of sufficient oxygen, the pyruvate produced by glycolysis goes into a second process called the *Krebs Cycle*.

■ The Krebs Cycle produces 36 new ATP molecules, and also waste products: carbon dioxide and water.

Pyruvate to Lactate

Now back to the pyruvate, standing at the crossroads. We've seen what happens when oxygen *is* present.

If oxygen *isn't* present, the pyruvate cannot go through the Krebs Cycle as it did in aerobic metabolism. Instead, it gets turned into **lactate**, also called lactic acid, as part of **anaerobic metabolism** (*anaerobic* because it takes place in the *absence* of oxygen).

This process does *not* produce any more ATP molecules.

So when you get to the end of anaerobic metabolism, your original glucose molecule has still only produced the two ATP molecules that were formed as the glucose became pyruvate.

Putting all three of these processes together, we get a completed picture that looks like this:

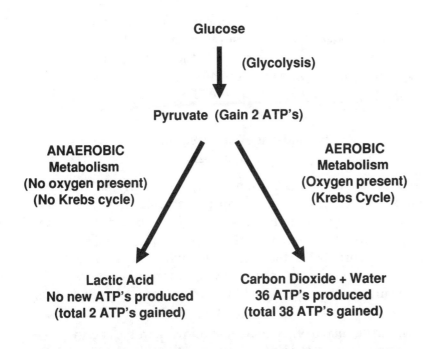

Glucose

(Glycolysis)

Pyruvate (Gain 2 ATP's)

ANAEROBIC	AEROBIC
Metabolism	**Metabolism**
(No oxygen present)	**(Oxygen present)**
(No Krebs cycle)	**(Krebs Cycle)**

Lactic Acid
No new ATP's produced
(total 2 ATP's gained)

Carbon Dioxide + Water
36 ATP's produced
(total 38 ATP's gained)

- If there isn't enough oxygen present to allow pyruvate to go through Krebs Cycle, it goes through a third process: *pyruvate-to-lactic acid.*

- The end product of pyruvate-to-lactic acid is *lactic acid* (also called *lactate*).

- Pyruvate-to-lactate does not produce any new ATP.

Just how do these four processes—ATP breakdown, glycolysis, Krebs Cycle, and pyruvate-to-lactate—relate to one another?

When you first begin to exercise, energy is supplied almost completely by the breakdown of ATP to ADP and phosphate. The muscles' initial ATP stores can be exhausted in as little as a fraction of a second by this energy mechanism, although this usually takes a couple of minutes.

First stage energy supplied by:
ATP → ADP + Phosphate

STAGES OF METABOLISM DURING EXERCISE

When muscle cells get the biochemical signal that more energy is needed than can be supplied by initial ATP stores, glycolysis begins. Because there is insufficient oxygen present at that time, the pyruvate must go into anaerobic metabolism—that is, no Krebs Cycle, only two ATP's per glucose molecule, and the production of *lactate*.

Second stage energy supplied by:
glycolysis

But lactate is *acidic* (it is, remember, lactic *acid*)—so when you produce lactate, you increase your muscle's acidity level (that is, lower the muscle's pH). Your muscle's capillaries—the very tiny blood vessels—are sensitive to pH. If the pH falls much *below* the norm of 7.4, the capillaries—which are normally closed—respond to the change by *opening up* to let more blood come in to the muscle. This blood brings more oxygen and carries away lactic acid, thereby helping restore the pH to 7.4.

The additional oxygen delivered allows aerobic energy production to proceed. The pyruvate produced in glycolysis can enter the Krebs Cycle, producing 36 new ATP's per glucose used.

Third stage energy supplied by:
Krebs Cycle

So during the initial few minutes of exercise, there are three phases of energy metabolism.

First, an **anaerobic** phase during which the muscle breaks down already-existing ATP to ADP and phosphate.

Second, another **anaerobic** phase, during which energy is produced via glycolysis—and as a result lactic acid accumulates and pH in muscle cells drops.

Third, a **mostly aerobic** phase. This starts after enough lactic acid has accumulated from anaerobic metabolism to cause enough of a pH drop to trigger opening of capillaries. With the opening of capillaries, new oxygen and glucose are delivered, and lactic acid is flushed out. There is now enough oxygen present for the Krebs cycle to provide substantial energy for the activity, although some anaerobic metabolism will continue.

Aerobic / Anaerobic Balance

Actually, all three energy production processes go on all the time. What changes is the relative contribution of each.

When you are at rest, the majority of energy is provided by the aerobic process. When you begin to exercise, you get the progression described above—breakdown of local ATP and glycolysis provide much of the energy while your cardio-vascular/respiratory system gets up to speed, then the aerobic process (including Krebs Cycle) provides more of the energy.

At this stage, how much energy is provided aerobically, and how much anaerobically depends on the length and intensity of the exercise. The anaerobic mechanism supplies most of the energy for extremely strenuous exercise of short duration—such as doing five reps of Bench Press with all the weight you can handle. The aerobic mechanism supplies much of the energy for low to moderate intensity exercise of extremely prolonged duration—such as running a marathon. While running, short speed bursts will temporarily increase the contribution of the anaerobic process.

■ Both aerobic and anaerobic energy processes go on side by side in the body all the time. What varies is the *relative contribution* of each—a balance controlled by exercise demand and amount of available oxygen.

■ Prolonged, low-intensity exercise—such as jogging—is primarily aerobic

■ High-intensity exercise—such as lifting heavy weights—is primarily anaerobic

Buffering

What happens to all the lactic acid produced by the anaerobic energy mechanism?

After being flushed out of the muscle tissue, it goes into the bloodstream where it makes the blood more acidic. Like the muscles, the blood functions best at a pH of 7.4, and, like the muscles, the blood has some *homeostatic* mechanisms to keep its pH balance normal.

One of these is its **buffering** ability.

Buffering involves converting an acidic substance into something that isn't so acidic.

Two compounds in the blood—**hemoglobin** (the same stuff that carries oxygen) and **bicarbonate**—are the primary buffers for lactic acid.

The end products of buffering by hemoglobin and bicarbonate are the same as the end products of aerobic energy production: carbon dioxide and water. It may come as a surprise, but it is actually the increase in carbon dioxide in your blood—and not the need for more oxygen—that triggers all the things associated with heavy exertion: faster heart rate, heavy breathing, faster blood circulation. All of these are intended to get the carbon dioxide from your blood to your lungs and out of your body as quickly as possible. Put another way, all are part of your body's homeostatic mechanism for controlling your acid/base balance (pH).

Eventually though, if you exercise long and hard enough, you overwhelm your body's ability to keep its pH at the proper level, even with your excellent buffering mechanisms. At that point, you stop exercising, because you feel too tired to continue.

- **Your body cannot tolerate large changes in pH (level of acidity).**

- **Several different processes *buffer* the lactic acid—act to keep the lactic acid from lowering the blood's pH.**

- **These processes turn the acid into carbon dioxide and water.**

- **Increased carbon dioxide in your blood makes you breathe harder (you get rid of the carbon dioxide by breathing it out).**

- **If you exercise long enough, or hard enough, the rate of production of lactic acid exceeds your body's ability to buffer that lactic acid; your blood pH drops, and you stop exercising because you feel too tired to continue.**

A while ago, we listed the sources of fuel for the three basic energy producing mechanisms in your body. These fuels are: ATP, circulating glucose, glycogen stored in muscles and in the liver, fat, and in some instances, protein. Having taken a good look at ATP, let's turn the spotlight on the roles of glycogen, fat, and protein.

GLUCOSE AND FAT

Recall that your body stores glucose as a polysaccharide called *glycogen*. Glycogen is stored in liver and muscle.

During the first few minutes of exercise, most of the energy for muscle contraction is derived from local *muscle glycogen* (which gets converted to glucose) and from glucose already circulating in the blood. As exercise continues, progressively more *liver glycogen* is converted to glucose, and is dispatched via the blood to the muscles. The longer and more intensely exercise continues, the more the glycogen stores diminish.

Glucose from Glycogen

Breakdown of glycogen is not the only means your body has of getting glucose for producing ATP. Your body can also make glucose from *protein* and *fat*; or, more specifically, from *amino acids* and the *glycerine part of fat molecules* (the part attached to the three fatty acids—see Chapter 6). The process of manufacturing new glucose is called **gluconeogenesis**.

Gluconeogenesis exacts a price for the glucose it generates, though. It temporarily reduces the body's protein "stores." In extreme cases, it can result in a significant reduction in lean body mass (muscle). This is the basis for the concept of **protein sparing**. Having sufficient glycogen reserves limits how much the body resorts to gluconeogenesis—and the breakdown of muscle—to provide needed glucose during prolonged exercise.

Glucose From Protein and Fat

■ Glycolysis, an essential part of the ATP-production process, requires glucose. Glucose is available from several sources:

❑ A certain amount is kept circulating in the blood (this is commonly referred to as *blood sugar*).

❏ Additional glucose is stored as *glycogen* in muscles and liver. As the body's glucose demand increases, the glycogen stored in the liver is converted to glucose, and is sent out into the bloodstream.

❏ As the body depletes its carbohydrate reserves, it can synthesize additional glucose from protein and from the glycerine part of fat molecules via a process called *gluconeogenesis*. Prolonged gluconeogenesis can result in a significant loss of muscle tissue.

Fat as an Energy Source

Gluconeogenesis is not the only way fat can act as a fuel for ATP production. In fact, during prolonged aerobic exercise, the *major* source of energy for ATP production is a fat-based process, called **fatty acid oxidation**.

Oxidation simply means to combine something with oxygen. So fatty acid oxidation is a process in which stored fat molecules break down and combine with oxygen.

Recall from Chapter 6 that fat molecules are **triglycerides**—glycerine with three long fatty acid chains attached. In the first phase of fat oxidation—called **lipolysis**—these long chains are snipped from the glycerine. The fatty acid chains, no longer attached to the glycerine, are now called *free* **fatty acids**.

The free fatty acids then enter the component of the cells responsible for energy production, the **mitochondria**, courtesy of a special transport carrier, **carnitine**.

Once inside the mitochondria, the free fatty acids are broken down into two-carbon fragments that bind to Coenzyme A. The resulting combination is called **acetyl-CoA**, which readily enters the Krebs Cycle to produce ATP.

■ Fat provides energy via a process called *fatty acid oxidation.*

■ Fatty acid oxidation is the primary energy production process during prolonged endurance exercise. It is our fourth energy production process, along with ATP breakdown, glycolysis, and the Krebs Cycle.

PRODUCING FUEL FOR ENERGY

All four energy production processes occur simultaneously during exercise.

However, the *limiting factor* for prolonged aerobic energy production is the availability of glycogen. When the body's glycogen stores are depleted, you have to stop exercising.*

You can do three things to push back the limit imposed by availability of glycogen:

■ Increase your glycogen storage capacity

■ Make sure your glycogen stores are full to capacity

■ Decrease the rate at which glycogen stores are depleted. (This requires increasing the contribution from fatty acid oxidation.)

What can you do to increase your glycogen storage capacity?

Exercise. Exercise itself appears to be the only way you can increase your glycogen storage *capacity*.

What can you do to make sure you actually store as much glycogen as you are capable of storing?

Eat the right foods. In general, that means making complex carbohydrates a large part of your diet. In particular, it means **carbo-loading** before an athletic event requiring endurance. Carbo-loading is discussed in greater detail in Chapter 20.

---

*Actually, you can continue, but only at a much-reduced level of energy production.

Glycogen Sparing

How about decreasing the rate at which glycogen stores are depleted?

Again, the solution is *exercise*. Endurance training has been shown to increase the contribution of fatty acid oxidation during endurance exercise. With more energy being derived from fatty acids, less needs to be derived from glycogen. The body's glycogen supplies are thus *spared* and last considerably longer.

■ The *limiting factor* for prolonged aerobic exercise is *glycogen storage*. When you run out of stored glycogen, you can continue only at a greatly reduced intensity level.

■ There are three ways to make your glycogen last as long as possible:

❑ *Increase storage capacity*. Regular endurance exercise increases the amount of glycogen you can store.

❑ *Store at or near capacity*. A diet high in complex carbohydrates, and the use of specialized techniques like carbo-loading, ensure that you store the maximum possible amount of glycogen.

❑ *Decrease the rate at which glycogen stores are depleted* by increasing the contribution by fatty acid oxidation. Your glycogen stores last longer if more of your required energy is supplied via fatty acid oxidation. Regular endurance exercise predisposes the body to rely more on fatty acid oxidation for energy.

To put all this energy theory into perspective, let's examine what happens, energy-wise, when you run:

You start running. As you begin moving the muscles in your arms and legs, you use the stored ATP almost immediately. The high-energy bonds in the ATP break apart, providing energy for muscle movement and producing ADP and phosphate. To keep moving your muscles, you need to generate new ATP.

For the moment—until reinforcements arrive—your muscles are low on oxygen. In the absence of oxygen, your glucose molecules (after becoming pyruvate) cannot go through the Krebs Cycle. Instead, you must rely primarily on anaerobic metabolism. Because anaerobic metabolism produces only two ATP molecules for each glucose molecule used (as opposed to the 38 ATP per glucose you get from aerobic metabolism), you have to burn up glucose much faster (nineteen times faster) to keep up the same level of energy.

As you push on, you continue to produce more lactic acid. The lactic acid diffuses out of your muscle cells and into the muscle capillaries, pushing your capillary pH down (making it more acidic). Your capillaries respond by opening up and allowing more blood to get through.

More blood means more oxygen, so aerobic metabolism— with its higher energy production—increases again. More blood also helps carry away lactic acid and restore the pH balance. So you now have reached a more comfortable state of exercise, in which the increased flow of blood helps compensate for the increased demands you are placing on your body.

How long you can continue in this more balanced state will depend on your level of cardiovascular/respiratory fitness. You may be able to continue for just a few minutes, or may last for two hours or more. The longer you continue to run, the more fat you oxidize and the more you draw from stores of glycogen in muscles and liver.

The harder and longer you run, the greater the percentage of total energy production will become anaerobic. Your natural buffering mechanisms will help control your pH balance, but at some point the lactic acid—produced by a growing proportion of anaerobic metabolism—will accumulate in quantities the buffering mechanisms can't control.

As this happens, you start to breathe a little faster. The acid is being turned into carbon dioxide and water; your faster breath-

ENERGY SUMMARY: WHAT HAPPENS WHEN YOU EXERCISE

ing helps expel the carbon dioxide and water, and keeps the lactic acid level under control.

But it's a losing battle. You keep breathing faster and harder, but the acidity keeps rising (pH keeps dropping). As proportionately more glucose gets channeled into anaerobic metabolism, you have to work harder to maintain your energy level at the same time you are producing more lactic acid.

Eventually, the production of acid overwhelms your body's ability to keep your pH at the proper level. At that point you are at the end of your endurance, and you have to stop.

Once you stop exercising, you recover quickly. You pant heavily, expelling carbon dioxide and water, which, several chemical reactions ago, used to be circulating acid. Some of the lactic acid floating around in your blood gets turned into pyruvate, and then goes on through the Krebs Cycle to produce energy.

At the same time, as the overall energy demand diminishes, the muscles re-establish higher levels of local oxygen, and aerobic metabolism dominates. This in turn reduces the level of lactate production, and your pH levels return to normal. Within a few minutes you are breathing normally and feeling fine.

SOME FINAL NOTES ON LACTIC ACID

Taking a step back from all the different energy mechanisms and fuels, there are two basic criteria for continued endurance performance:

- Your body needs a constant supply of glucose for energy.
- Your body must deal with the inevitable buildup of lactic acid.

We've already discussed maximizing your glycogen stores. Now, let's see what you can do to deal with lactic acid.

How quickly lactic acid ends your exercising depends on three things:

- your buffering ability
- the vascularity of your muscles
- your ability to tolerate a low pH

Can you improve your buffering ability?

Maybe. Remember that the two main buffering compounds in your blood are bicarbonate and hemoglobin. You can increase the bicarbonate in your blood by taking bicarbonate, such as drinking a solution of sodium bicarbonate and water (Arm & Hammer, right out of the kitchen cupboard). There is some research to indicate that taking bicarbonate before an aerobic event may improve endurance.

The other buffering compound is hemoglobin, the oxygen-carrying component of blood. You can increase the amount of hemoglobin in your blood by blood doping (see Chapter 12) or by moving to a high altitude.

The improvements in endurance seen with blood doping are usually attributed to increased oxygen carrying capacity, but there may be a component of increased buffering capacity as well. (This is obviously a more extreme measure than drinking a bicarbonate solution.)

Muscular vascularity also increases endurance. If you have more blood vessels, more oxygen can be delivered, and proportionately less anaerobic metabolism will take place. That means less lactic acid will be produced, and the lactic acid that *is* produced will be taken away from the muscle cells faster.

Can you increase your muscular vascularity through diet? No. But you can through exercise. Regular endurance exercise can actually increase the number of capillaries in your muscles, and thereby increase your endurance.

The ability to tolerate a low pH increases endurance. For reasons that are not clear, athletes who consistently exercise are able to tolerate levels of lactic acid in their blood that non-athletes cannot. High levels of lactic acid cause muscle pain and fatigue, and athletes are able to withstand this pain and fatigue more easily than are non-athletes. Clearly, being able to tolerate muscle pain and fatigue can give an athlete extra endurance.

The only way to develop this tolerance is through regular exercise.

This, then, is the physiological explanation for something you've known all along: if you exercise regularly, your endurance improves dramatically. This once again points to the importance of establishing and maintaining a regular exercise program in conjunction with any nutritional undertaking. Only when both approaches function in harmony can you achieve peak athletic performance.

■ **You can push back the limitations on aerobic performance imposed by lactic acid buildup by:**

❑ **enhancing buffering capacity**

❑ **increasing muscular vascularity**

❑ **raising lactic acid tolerance level**

■ **All three goals can be accomplished through regular endurance training.**

■ **There is some evidence that buffering capacity can be increased by taking sodium bicarbonate before endurance events.**

❖   ❖   ❖

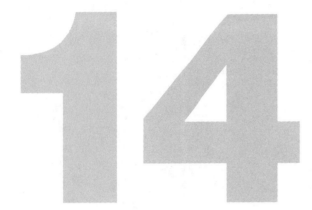

WATER AND SPORTS DRINKS

Water is the most critical nutrient for athletic performance. Most nutrients—even essential ones—can be absent from your diet for days or even weeks without causing really serious problems. But your body's water supply must be replenished frequently. This chapter explores the role of water in athletic performance, and the use of sports drinks to maintain optimum fluid and electrolyte balance during prolonged exercise.

WATER—THE TEMPERATURE CONTROL SYSTEM

You are about 60% water by weight. So if you weigh 160 pounds, your body contains about 96 pounds (12 gallons) of water, only a gallon of which is in your blood.

■ Two-thirds of your total body water is inside your cells, and is called **intracellular fluid**.

■ The remaining one-third is outside cells, and is called **extracellular fluid**. Most of the extracellular fluid surrounds cells. Only a small part (one-twelfth of the total body water) is in blood in the form of **plasma**.

Water performs a number of vitally important functions.

It provides an appropriate environment for your body's many chemical reactions, and for diffusion of nutrients into cells and wastes out of cells. In the form of plasma, water serves as the internal transportation system among organs, delivering nutrients and clearing wastes.

Most important to the athlete, however, is water's function as the regulator of **body temperature**. Exercise generates heat, and this heat must be gotten rid of for exercise to continue. This is why water is critical to athletic performance—your ability to get rid of heat during exercise depends mostly on the formation and evaporation of sweat, and sweat requires water.

During prolonged exercise you can lose a *lot* of water through sweat; if you lose enough water without replacing it, you compromise your performance: A loss of 2% of body weight through sweating does not significantly impair athletic performance, but does impair temperature regulation. A loss of 3% of body weight through sweating reduces muscle endurance. A loss of 4 to 6% reduces both muscle endurance and muscle strength. A loss of more than 6% may cause severe heat cramps, heat exhaustion, heat stroke, coma, and death.

Nutrients in Sweat

Two nutrients—**sodium** and **chloride**—are lost in significant quantities through sweating. Significantly, sodium and chloride are the two elements primarily responsible for maintaining appropriate water content in the interstitial fluid (the water around the cells) and in the blood plasma.

You might expect, then, that heavy sweating would lead to a deficiency of sodium and chloride in your blood plasma and interstitial fluid, and that replacing sodium and chloride would be the appropriate action. Oddly enough, just the opposite is true—**heavy sweating *increases* the *concentrations* of sodium and chloride in your body's fluids; what you need to replace is *water*.**

How can this be?

When you sweat, you lose water, sodium, and chloride, but you lose proportionately *more* water. The body water left behind ends up having proportionately *more* sodium and chloride than it did to start with. So, after sweating, the *amounts* of water, sodium, and chloride are all decreased, but the *concentration* of sodium and chloride remaining in your body is *increased*.

The amounts of sodium and chloride lost—while significant—are usually not large enough to require replacement during anything less than marathon-length exercise. Likewise, the small amounts of potassium, magnesium, and other minerals lost in sweat are not lost in quantities sufficient to require replenishment during exercise.

Fluid Intake During Exercise

Water is a different story, though. It is essential that you drink fluids during prolonged exercise to prevent dehydration.

Dehydration causes...

- **water to be removed from inside cells** (intracellular fluid), so the chemical reactions are no longer taking place in an optimum environment

- **water to be removed from around cells** (extracellular fluid), possibly impairing diffusion of nutrients into cells and wastes away from cells

- **a drop in blood volume**, forcing the heart to pump harder, and thereby increasing the stress on the heart

- **a decrease in water available for sweat**, interfering with heat dissipation, and in turn, compromising performance

Dehydration, and its negative effects on performance, are easily prevented by drinking appropriate fluids during prolonged exertion.

- **Water's most important function for athletes is regulating body temperature, via sweating.**

- **A water loss amounting to only 3% of bodyweight reduces muscular endurance.**

- **A water loss amounting to 4% to 6% reduces both muscular endurance and strength.**

- **Dehydration not only impairs athletic performance but poses a serious health risk.**

■ You lose sodium and chloride as well as water when you sweat, but you lose proportionately more water, leaving you with *higher* concentrations of sodium and chloride in your blood. So what you primarily need to replenish during exercise is *water*.

❑ Prolonged exercise (such as running a marathon) performed in extreme heat may create a need for electrolyte (sodium and chloride) replacement during exercise.

❑ Potassium, magnesium, iron, and other minerals are also lost in sweat, but not in quantities sufficient to require replenishment during exercise.

SPORTS DRINKS

Sports drinks refers to preparations that athletes drink during exercise. These are usually commercially produced. The basic goal of sports drinks is to replace water lost through sweating. Secondary goals include replacement of electrolytes lost through sweating, and provision of additional energy fuel (carbohydrate, usually in the form of glucose) to spare muscle and liver glycogen stores and prolong endurance.

What to Drink

Much research has centered on determining a formulation for sports drinks that will get the water and other ingredients into your bloodstream in minimum time. Two major factors affect that time: gastric emptying rate, and rate of intestinal absorption.

Gastric Emptying Rate

Gastric emptying rate refers to the speed with which the contents of the stomach empty into the small intestine, where they can be absorbed. A number of factors affect gastric emptying rate, including:

Volume. The greater the amount of stomach contents, the faster those contents enter the small intestine. This factor has little impact on design of sports drinks. Any drink consumed in large enough quantities to bring volume-accelerated emptying into play would leave the athlete feeling bloated, and most likely would interfere with sports performance.

Caloric Content. The higher the caloric content, the slower the gastric emptying rate. Caloric content seems to be the most important factor influencing gastric emptying rate. This has led some researchers to suggest that glucose and other forms of carbohydrate be left out of sports drinks because they retard emptying time. Inclusion of these substances, they hypothesize, might slow absorption of fluid enough to interfere with optimum sports performance.

However, current research indicates that under exercise conditions, plain water and a ten percent (or less) carbohydrate solution exhibit similar emptying rates.

Osmolarity. This term refers to the *concentration* of particles in a given amount of fluid. For example, a cup of water with three teaspoons of sugar has a higher osmolarity than a cup of water with one teaspoon of sugar.

For many years, higher osmolarities were thought to slow gastric emptying. However, higher-osmolarity drinks are usually higher in calories as well, and researchers now believe the higher caloric values, not the difference in osmolarity, have been responsible for the slower emptying rate demonstrated in many studies.

Intestinal Absorption

The second major factor affecting the time required for the ingredients of a sports drink to get into the athlete's blood is the **rate of intestinal absorption**.

Studies show that water is absorbed much more quickly in the presence of both glucose and sodium.

In fact, although glucose slows gastric emptying, **the benefits that glucose provides by hastening intestinal absorption and providing extra endurance *fuel* outweigh the drawbacks of slowed gastric emptying time.** This is the basis for the first guideline of what to drink during prolonged exercise: the beverage should include some carbohydrate.

Many studies demonstrate that consuming carbohydrate during exercise effectively increases endurance. The best type of carbohydrate to include in sports drinks remains controversial.

Glucose polymers. Glucose polymers are long chains of glucose molecules (or *polysaccharides*; see Chapter 6). Since the glucose molecules in glucose polymers are all tied up in long glucose polymer chains, the osmolarity (particle concentration) of a glucose-polymer drink is *low*, even though the calorie content is *high*. This has led some manufacturers to use ***glucose polymers*** in their sports drinks, based on the thinking that the lower osmolarity will increase the gastric emptying rate, improving the efficacy of the drink.

Research indicates this is not the case. Ingestion of a glucose polymer solution during exercise results in similar times for gastric emptying and intestinal absorption as does ingestion of an equal- calorie, equal-volume glucose solution. This means that glucose polymer solutions are no more effective than straight glucose solutions at getting fluid into your bloodstream quickly.

Fructose. Fructose stimulates slightly less intestinal water absorption than the same concentration glucose solution, and thus is slightly less effective at getting the fluid into your bloodstream quickly.

Also, high-concentration fructose solutions have been shown to cause gastrointestinal distress and diarrhea, both during rest and exercise, diminishing the attractiveness of fructose as a carbohydrate source in sports drinks.

Sucrose. Sucrose is rapidly broken down in the small intestine to glucose and fructose. The fructose portion is associated with slightly less water absorption, as indicated above. So sucrose is a slightly less-effective carbohydrate to include in sports drinks than glucose.

The second guideline: the best carbohydrates to include in sports drink are glucose, glucose polymer, and sucrose, in that order.

Carbohydrate Type

Sweat contains small quantities of sodium, potassium, and other minerals important for fluid balance. Losses of these minerals, called ***electrolytes***, through sweating normally pose no

Electrolyte Content

threat either to health or performance. A post-exercise meal replenishes all electrolyte losses.

However, performance of extreme endurance events—triathlons, marathons—in the heat may necessitate some electrolyte supplementation during exercise. Electrolyte supplementation can:

- replace electrolytes lost through sweating and thus help maintain the body's electrolyte and fluid balance
- prevent onset of **hyponatremia** (abnormally low blood sodium concentration) brought on by replenishing major sweat losses with water alone

Let's expand on that second point a bit. As previously explained, water losses do outweigh electrolyte losses during exercise, resulting in higher electrolyte concentrations in the blood, and a greater need to replenish water than to replenish electrolytes. However, it's possible to end up with *too low* a concentration of electrolytes in your blood if, during extremely prolonged exercise, you drink a really large quantity of plain water to replenish fluid losses. Using a fluid-replacement drink containing a low concentration of electrolytes will prevent this problem.

Inclusion of small amounts of electrolytes in sports drinks also has other benefits, including:

- increasing the absorption of water in the small intestine
- increasing the palatability of the solution, raising the likelihood that you will drink enough to meet fluid requirements of heavy exercise

Third guideline: Sports drinks for use during prolonged endurance exercise should contain low concentrations of electrolytes, including sodium, potassium, and chloride.

What to Drink: The Bottom Line

For exercise up to four hours, the only real requirement is water. Over four hours, your sports drink should include low concentrations of electrolytes.

Also, for any continuous exercise over one hour, drinking a sports drink which contains carbohydrate (preferably glucose, glucose polymer, or sucrose) may increase your endurance.

How Much to Drink

We pointed out that large volumes of fluid—a pint or more—empty faster from the stomach than smaller amounts. However, such large amounts are impractical to drink during athletic competition. They can make you feel bloated, and may interfere with optimum performance.

A better amount seems to be about 150 to 250 milliliters (roughly six ounces).

How Often to Drink

You should drink about six ounces every ten to fifteen minutes during prolonged exercise (anything over half an hour). *Don't rely on thirst* to tell you how much to drink. Thirst is a poor indicator of fluid needs—if you rely on thirst, you won't drink enough.

A Final Caution: Salt Tablets

It used to be common for athletes to take salt tablets when exercising in hot weather. The belief was that since salt was lost in sweat, it should be replaced to keep the body's water and electrolytes in balance. This belief contains a grain of truth, at least for prolonged endurance exercise (as explained above), but using salt tablets to replenish electrolyte losses is not the right solution.

A *low*-concentration solution of sodium and other electrolytes, such as is found in most commercial sports drinks, is the best way to address electrolyte losses. The high concentration of sodium and chloride from salt tablets is dangerous overkill that increases the load on your kidneys, can cause nausea and vomiting, and can accelerate dehydration. Stay away from these!

■ **Guidelines for water replenishment during exercise:**

❑ For events over one-half hour, drink approximately 6 ounces of water (or sports beverage) every ten to fifteen minutes.

❑ Don't rely on thirst to tell you when and how much to drink. Thirst is a poor indicator of fluid needs.

❑ For events up to four hours in length, water is an adequate replenishment drink. For events over four hours, a replenishment drink containing low concentrations of electrolytes is preferable.

❑ A sports drink containing up to a 10% concentration of carbohydrate (preferably as glucose, glucose polymer, or sucrose), will increase endurance without slowing gastric emptying time.

❑ *Don't take salt tablets!* They exacerbate the problem of increased sodium and chloride concentrations caused by sweating, put a strain on your kidneys, may cause nausea and vomiting, and can accelerate dehydration.

❖   ❖   ❖

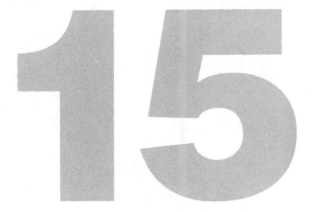

WEIGHT CONTROL AND BODY COMPOSITION

Most serious athletes want to put on or take off weight at some point in their athletic careers. Bodybuilders continually strive to increase muscle mass. Wrestlers may *have* to lose (or gain) weight to meet weigh-in requirements. And even the weekend athlete may want to gain or lose a few pounds in the quest for fitness and improved appearance.

This chapter reviews the principles of weight gain and loss.

LOSING WEIGHT

Weight loss occurs when calories consumed are insufficient to meet the body's energy requirements. You can achieve this goal by eating less, exercising more, or by doing both of these.

In any case, the goal is to lose *fat*, not muscle. Although any significant drop in weight will be accompanied by some muscle loss, certain weight loss practices can keep lean tissue loss to a minimum. These include:

■ restricting caloric intake but continuing to eat a balanced diet

■ avoiding extreme calorie-restricting techniques such as fasting

■ continuing to exercise during periods of caloric restriction

Weight loss should not exceed one to two pounds a week. Although individual metabolism varies, a deficit of 1,000 calories a day should be sufficient to lose that amount. (Each pound of fat loss represents 3,500 calories utilized. Seven days times 1,000 calories = 7,000 cal., or two lbs. of fat utilized per week.)

GAINING WEIGHT

Gaining weight requires consuming more calories than necessary to meet your body's energy demands.

Clearly, you don't just want to gain *weight*—you want to gain *muscle*. Extra bodyfat *decreases* speed and endurance. And for bodybuilders, gaining extra fat is obviously counterproductive.

Increasing muscle mass requires:

- muscular overload, such as that provided by a progressive weight training program. **You cannot increase muscle mass by dietary manipulation alone.**

- sufficient dietary calories to support the energy demands both of training and of the muscle building process

- a *very slight* increase in protein over what the sedentary person requires. **This does not mean you need to increase your protein consumption.** As explained in Chapter 4, most athletes are already getting at least twice as much protein as is needed to meet the increased demand imposed by muscle growth. Eating still more protein will make you fat, not bigger.

Gaining muscle requires walking a fine caloric line between consuming too few calories and consuming too many. Too few will not supply sufficient energy for muscle growth. Too many will increase the amount of fat stored. As a general rule, adding about 750 to 900 calories a day to your *stable weight* diet should promote muscle gains of as much as a pound a week. If that sounds slow, imagine weighing forty to fifty pounds more in a year than you do right now—all of it muscle!

THE PSYCHOLOGY OF WEIGHT CONTROL

Few aspects of sports take more self-control and patience than weight control. Athletes are willing to train for hours a day, for years on end, to develop the skills required for top performance, but they often have great difficulty controlling their eating habits and making appropriate weight gains or losses. Ask an athlete to train an extra hour and he or she will probably be willing. Ask an athlete to eat less ice cream and he or she may feel deprived.

The psychological side of weight control is very important, but beyond the scope of this book. If you have a great deal of trouble setting weight-related goals and following through on them, you may want to look at some of the excellent books on the psychological aspects of body weight,* or talk to one the many counselors trained in the complexities of this area. Getting past a psychological *sticking point* is sometimes the change that makes weight control—and peak athletic performance—possible.

■ Weight loss requires creating a *negative energy balance* (more calories out than in).

■ Weight loss should not exceed one to two pounds per week.

■ The optimum weight loss program...

❑ restricts caloric intake, but provides a balanced diet

❑ does not include extreme calorie-restricting techniques such as fasting

❑ relies on a combination of diet plus exercise to achieve a caloric deficit

*Health For Life's *Psychology of Weight Loss* program addresses this subject in detail.

■ **Weight (muscle) gain requires a slightly positive energy balance, but more important, it requires *exercise*. Muscles only grow if overloaded.**

❑ *Weight gain does not require increased dietary protein unless your diet is protein-deficient to begin with (See Chapter 4)*

❑ **A caloric overload of 750 to 900 calories a day will result in weight gain of about one pound per week, given sufficient exercise stimulus.**

BODY COMPOSITION

Body composition refers to the relative amounts of fat and lean tissue in the body, and is usually expressed as **percentage bodyfat**—that is, as a number indicating what percent of total body weight is fat.

For many athletes, body composition is as important as weight. The bodybuilder, for example, relies on a low percentage bodyfat to look ripped. Likewise, the marathoner maintains a low percentage bodyfat to minimize the extra baggage he or she carries for twenty-six miles of running.

Lowering bodyfat requires a calorie-restricted but balanced diet coupled with adequate exercise. **Protein-only**, and **carbohydrate-only** diets, two popular methods for lowering bodyfat, are not effective for achieving that end and can be dangerous to your health. The protein-only diet puts excessive strain on the kidneys. The carbohydrate-only diet does not supply the amino acids the body needs, forcing the body to enter a **catabolic** state, where amino acids required for the body's maintenance are obtained by breaking down lean muscle tissue. Prolonged adherence to a carbohydrate-only diet can result in a substantial loss of lean tissue.

How Lean is Lean?

For reference, fit adult men average sixteen to eighteen percent bodyfat; fit adult women, twenty-four to twenty-six percent.

Serious competitive athletes generally have lower numbers.

Male endurance athletes may have as little as five to seven percent bodyfat; women, seven to ten percent. These figures represent rock bottom. Lower bodyfat percentages are incompatible with basic good health, and may harm performance.

The bottom line: **There is no magic bodyfat percentage that guarantees peak performance.** However, in weight-matched sports in which athletes compete against others in the same weight class—such as wrestling and weightlifting—the athlete with the lower percentage of bodyfat has a competitive advantage, all other things being equal.

Measuring Body Composition

A number of methods exist for measuring body composition.

Hydrostatic Weighing

The most accurate way to measure body composition is by **hydrostatic weighing**, also called **underwater weighing**.

With this method, the athlete is first weighed conventionally, and then weighed while submerged in a large vat of water.

Since fat is less dense than lean tissue, a person with more body fat will be less dense, and will weigh proportionately less underwater. The difference between what a person weighs out of water and what he or she weighs in water can be used to calculate what percentage of that person's weight is fat.

Impedance Testing

This method takes advantage of the fact that fat conducts electricity differently from muscle. Electrodes are attached to hands and feet and a small electric current is passed through the body (this doesn't hurt). The amount of resistance encountered by the current gives an indication of the total bodyfat.

Infrared

This brand-new method relies on the fact that fat transmits infrared light differently from muscle. Special infrared-producing and infrared-receiving pads are attached to the biceps. A beam of infrared light is then passed through the arm. The amount of light emerging from the arm is used by the device to to determine the subject's total bodyfat.

Calipers

The least-expensive method of measuring body composition is to use a skin-pinching device, called **skinfold calipers**.

This instrument, available through surgical supply outlets, is used to measure skinfold thickness at the triceps, scapular (shoulder blade) and iliac crest (hip) regions. Conversion tables, tailored to sex and age, allow you to convert these measurements into overall percentages of bodyfat.

■ **For optimal athletic performance, body composition—relative amounts of fat and lean tissue in the body—is as important as weight.**

■ **In weight-matched events, the athlete with the lower percentage of bodyfat will have a competitive advantage, all other things being equal.**

■ **Body Composition references:**

    ❑ **For fitness, adult males: 16 to 18% bodyfat; adult females: 24 to 26% bodyfat.**

    ❑ **For endurance competition: lower than the fitness levels, but no lower than...males: 5 to 7%; females: 7 to 10%.**

❖   ❖   ❖

16

ERGOGENIC AIDS

The term *ergogenic aid* refers to any substance or process that enhances your ability to do physical work. (*Ergo* comes from the Greek word *ergon*, meaning *work*; *genic* means *producing*.)

Without question, the greatest ergogenic aid is **exercise**. Improvements in strength and endurance are usually quite dramatic, often exceeding fifty percent, in sedentary individuals who begin to exercise regularly. But when most people speak of ergogenic aids, they are usually referring to that seemingly endless variety of substances—from bee pollen to octacosanol—that athletes take to get a competitive edge.

Do any of these substances work?

THE ERGOGENIC POSSIBILITIES

There are only four ways *any* substance might improve your ability to produce work. These involve the way the body stores energy, utilizes energy, and translates energy into physical movement.

An ergogenic aid might:

■ add to your body's energy stores, and therefore prolong endurance by increasing the amount of available fuel

■ improve your metabolism of fuel, so you use that fuel more efficiently

- improve your endurance by slowing the accumulation of the fatigue-causing by-products of energy metabolism
- enhance your nervous system's ability to coordinate your muscle fibers, and thereby increase your physical strength

Actually, there is a *fifth* way an ergogenic aid might work—it might make you *think* your performance will be improved. It is an established scientific fact the mind can create physiological effects in the body based on a person's belief that a particular substance or practice will produce a certain physiological effect, even if the substance is in fact physiologically inert. This phenomenon is called the **placebo effect**. Athletes have been made to run faster, jump higher, and lift heavier weights after being given sugar pills and being told those pills were some incredible new performance drug. Likewise, doctors have cured all manner of ills, and psychiatrists have changed all manner of behaviors, using essentially empty capsules accompanied by a convincing line.

In fact, almost *anything* can improve performance if you believe it will. In this chapter, however, we'll limit our consideration to ergogenic aids which *do* have (or are at least *purported* to have) demonstrable physiological effects based on their biochemical activity, not on the placebo effect.

This chapter is not intended to be exhaustive. Far too many substances are claimed to have ergogenic qualities to explore them all here. Instead, we will focus on some of the more popular substances (many of which don't actually do anything), as well as some of the lesser known, but potentially more effective, options.

POSSIBILITY #1: MORE FUEL

Recall from Chapter 13 that your body stores energy as glycogen in your liver and muscles, and as fat in various fat deposits around your body. These energy stores are enough to see you through two to three hours of exercise, but after that, your diminishing glycogen reserves limit your endurance.

So, theoretically, one way a substance could enhance your athletic performance would be to provide extra fuel. Let's look at a few of the substances that might fall in this category.

Chemical Fuels: CP and ATP

Adenosine triphosphate (ATP) and the related compound creatine phosphate (CP) are the final links in the chain of energy production. Each stores small amounts of energy in its chemical bonds, and supplies the energy to make your muscles move. As soon as you start working your muscles, your ATP and CP concentrations decline dramatically. Some athletes have extrapolated from this fact that they might improve their performance by either taking ATP and CP orally or injecting them into specific muscles.

Neither method works, for two reasons:

First, the concentrations of these substances in the muscles fibers are not increased as by supplementation.

Second, even though the concentrations decline during exercise, the muscles do not become ATP-depleted; instead, the decline triggers increased carbohydrate metabolism, which keeps the muscle supplied with newly-synthesized ATP.

So although it is appealing to think supplementary ATP and CP might supply extra muscle fuel, the truth is they don't.

Carbohydrates

Wait a minute—what are carbohydrates doing in a chapter on ergogenic aids? Well, remember that an ergogenic aid is something that enables you to produce more work—and right now we're looking for substances that might supply extra fuel. The number one ergogenic in this category is carbohydrates.

As explained in the *Energy and Endurance* chapter, when you consume a diet high in complex carbohydrates, you store greater-than- usual amounts of glycogen in your muscles and liver. The stored glycogen is *fuel*, and the more of it you have the longer you can work. So carbohydrates have a significant ergogenic potential.

This potential can be maximized, for short periods of time, through carbo-loading (as discussed in Chapter 22). Carbo-loading enables you to store glycogen in even larger amounts than you would if you simply followed a high-carbohydrate diet. These increased stores are definitely ergogenic—that is, they provide even larger amounts of fuel and so increase your ability to produce work.

Finally, carbohydrates can increase your endurance if you take them during prolonged exercise (exercise in excess of one hour). When consumed as part of a carefully-prepared beverage (see Chapter 14), carbohydrates can raise your blood glucose level. Your muscles can then use this added glucose as fuel. This helps your glycogen stores last a little longer, increasing your endurance.

So ergogenic aids do not have to be exotic to work. We *expect* them to be because so many exotic-sounding products are *marketed* as ergogenic aids. But carbohydrates are a perfect illustration that informed and disciplined use of ordinary nutrients can be ergogenic.

Fat is an important source of energy. Your body stores much more energy as fat than as carbohydrate. The relative amounts of carbohydrates and fat you use as fuel vary constantly during different phases of exercise.

The more you burn fat, the less you have to burn glycogen; the longer the glycogen lasts, the longer you can keep going during prolonged exercise. So anything that increases the contribution fat oxidation makes to muscular energy production should increase your endurance.

Recall that your body uses fat for energy in the form of *free fatty acids*, which circulate in your blood. This fact has led some theoreticians to speculate that endurance could be increased by finding a way to *increase* the free fatty acids in the athlete's blood.

The concept is simple: If you have more fatty acids in your blood, your muscles can use more fatty acids for energy. You therefore will use less glycogen. And you will thus have greater endurance.

Sounds logical enough.

So how do you increase the free fatty acids in your blood? Generally speaking, in only one way: with caffeine. A second way, invoking the **fight-or-flight response**, works but isn't really under voluntary control.

Caffeine, used carefully, can safely increase the level of free fatty acids in your blood, with some accompanying ergogenic effect. We will discuss caffeine in more detail in a moment.

The **fight-or-flight** response, what your body calls upon in times of danger, *naturally increases* the free fatty acids in your blood.

This happens because the fight-or-flight response causes the release of hormones called *catecholamines*, such as epinephrine (adrenaline). Catecholamines stimulate both the breakdown of

Free Fatty Acids

fat molecules and the breakdown of glycogen, but stimulate the breakdown of fat molecules *more*.

As a result, fat oxidation increases, which may prolong glycogen stores in the long run, enhancing endurance. This may even occur to some extent as a result of normal nervousness or excitement. So when you get nervous before a big event—especially an endurance event—don't be concerned: your nervousness may mean extra energy a couple of hours down the line!

POSSIBILITY #2: BETTER METABOLISM

The amount of energy you produce, as well as the overall effect on your endurance, varies according to both the *kind* of energy-producing metabolism taking place (aerobic or anaerobic) and the particular *fuel* being broken down (glycogen or fat). Since these factors affect how efficiently you produce energy during exercise, it stands to reason that if you could find ways to *influence* those factors, you would also be able to influence energy production and endurance.

Certain ergogenics *do* promote improvements in endurance by altering metabolism. This section looks at the plusses and minuses of using these substances.

Caffeine

Caffeine is not as benign an ergogenic aid as, say, complex carbohydrates—caffeine is a drug.

What does caffeine *do* to your body? It:

- stimulates your central nervous system; this is what increases alertness, and makes some people jittery
- stimulates the kidneys to produce more urine; this is what causes the well-known increase in trips to the bathroom after a cup of coffee
- increases respiratory rate
- may enhance the strength of contracting muscle

These changes are more prominent in people who do not habitually consume caffeine; in fact, many of these changes are not seen at all in habitual caffeine users.

Although study results are not unanimous, general consensus holds that caffeine improves endurance performance. It appears to accomplish this through at least three mechanisms.

First, and probably most significant, caffeine causes something similar to the **fight-or-flight response—it stimulates the** release of catecholamines, which in turn stimulate fat break-down and bring about an increase in fatty acid oxidation. The net result is a relative sparing of glycogen, and increased endurance.

Second, caffeine may affect the *intensity* of exercise. In some studies, athletes taking caffeine have been found to perform at higher levels of intensity than athletes taking a placebo. How caffeine accomplishes this is not known; it may be that caffeine raises the maximum intensity level you can *tolerate* during pro-longed exercise. Because tolerance is increased, your maximum effort may take you to a higher level of intensity.

Third, caffeine may influence performance through its *psychological* effects. Caffeine stimulates the central nervous system. The psychological resulting lift may cause you not to tire as quickly, and to feel less muscular effort in general. Caffeine may also stimulate clear and alert thinking, which could enhance athletic performance in more subtle ways.

How much caffeine is the right amount for achieving these effects?

The best current estimate is approximately 250 to 300 milli-grams—about the amount in two cups of coffee—taken a little while before beginning prolonged exercise. See the table below for the caffeine content of various sources.

If you're thinking of using caffeine as an ergogenic aid, re-member that only in prolonged endurance situations is caffeine likely to help you. **Other than its potential psychological effects, none of the benefits of caffeine are available during short-term exercise.**

Also, because of caffeine's diuretic effect (stimulation of the kidneys), you are much more likely to become dehydrated

SELECTED SOURCES OF CAFFEINE

SOURCE	MG. OF CAFFEINE (approx.)
Coffee (1 cup)	208
Black Tea (1 cup)	60
Cola (12 ounces)	40
Chocolate (1 ounce)	35
Decaf Coffee (1 cup)	6

having taken caffeine. This can seriously jeopardize performance.

Will caffeine hurt you?

In recent years investigators have disagreed strongly about caffeine's possible negative effects. However, certain conclusions seem to be gaining more general acceptance.

Small amounts of caffeine—one or two cups of coffee a day—probably won't hurt you.

This is *not* to say a small amount of caffeine will have no *effect*, because it surely will. Rather, the effects at that level of intake should be more or less limited to the immediate stimulation, and should not cause some of the other, more harmful effects that caffeine *can* cause.

As noted in Chapter 12, caffeine may, when taken in larger amounts, cause anxiety, heart palpitations, nervousness, irritability, insomnia, nausea, diarrhea, and headaches. Injected in large amounts, it can even cause convulsions. Caffeine may also increase risk of heart attack, cancer, and fibrocystic breast disease, but these associations remain controversial.

Caffeine is a diuretic, stimulating the kidneys to produce urine. This partially dehydrates you, and it only takes a little dehydration to limit your ability to achieve peak performance.

A regular caffeine user develops a tolerance for the drug, and therefore will be less affected by taking it than will be someone who does not have it regularly. The maximum effect seems to be realized when the user has not had caffeine for at least four days.

Finally, ergogenic properties aside, caffeine does nothing positive for your health.

At the very best, it may improve your endurance by a small amount without doing you any physical harm. However, it may cause some of the physical problems mentioned above—any *one* of which could hurt your athletic performance.

Psychomotor Stimulants

Psychomotor stimulants include *amphetamines, cocaine,* and generally anything you might think of as *speed*. These drugs, which produce strong feelings of confidence and well-being, have become very popular among both athletes and non-athletes (see Chapter 12).

Psychomotor stimulants do appear to have several ergogenic effects. They:

■ may increase aerobic endurance

■ may decrease recovery time following work

■ may work much like caffeine to increase fat oxidation and thus conserve glycogen during prolonged exercise

■ may improve reaction times in athletes who are already tired

■ can increase muscular strength

Against the potential benefits just listed, you have to weigh the potential harm—and the potential harm is extreme.

Physical risks include heart problems, high blood pressure, gastrointestinal disturbances, insomnia, digestive difficulties, and sexual dysfunction. Athletes have been known to die from heat exhaustion when psychomotor stimulants prevented them from recognizing their body's warnings against overexertion.

Psychological risks include apathy, intense depression, paranoia and psychosis.

Because psychomotor stimulants are generally very addictive, problems developing from their use may be difficult to get rid of.

POSSIBILITY #3: FEWER BY-PRODUCTS

Recall from Chapter 13 that after you reach the point during exercise—a minute or two after starting—at which oxygen reinforcements have arrived, the biggest single factor in the onset of fatigue will be your pH balance.

As you continue to produce lactic acid through anaerobic metabolism, your body has to work harder and harder to keep your pH balance normal.

Eventually you reach a point at which your body can no longer keep your pH at the proper level. That's when you stop exercising, because you feel exhausted.*

Since the build-up of these by-products of energy metabolism—most notably lactic acid—brings on fatigue and exhaustion, it seems logical that a substance which would slow the accumulation of those by-products might increase endurance.

This section examines a couple of substances whose ergogenic potential is based on this possibility.

---

*The exact mechanism limiting muscular exertion is not known. This explanation reflects current thinking on the subject.

Sodium Bicarbonate

One of the ways your body **buffers** the accumulation of lactic acid is by releasing bicarbonate. Why not beat your body to the punch, then, and take sodium bicarbonate (baking soda) orally prior to exercising?

Although the gains are small, sodium bicarbonate *does* appear to prolong endurance when taken prior to exercise. It does this by inducing *alkalosis*—a state of increased alkalinity—which in effect gives your body an **acid deficit** at the beginning of exercise.

In a state of alkalosis, your body can neutralize a greater amount of acid. Since acid build-up brings on fatigue and exhaustion, neutralizing more acid slows the build-up and prolongs endurance.

Taking sodium bicarbonate appears to improve performance not only in prolonged aerobic exercise but also in short, high-intensity exercise as well.

In one experiment, experienced runners given 21 grams of sodium bicarbonate (the equivalent of 10.5 Alka Seltzers) over two hours ran an average of 2.9 seconds faster in an 800 meter race. It may not sound like much, but a 2.9 second improvement translates into a distance of 19 meters, which can easily be the difference between first and last place in an 800 meter race. Furthermore, although they didn't know if they had taken the sodium bicarbonate or a placebo, those who took the sodium bicarbonate felt they had not done well because they *had too much left at the finish line*.

Although they might not have known prior to the race whether they had gotten sodium bicarbonate or a placebo, half of them found out soon after. Approximately three hours after taking the sodium bicarbonate, the runners experienced what the researchers delicately described as *urgent diarrhea*.

The long-term consequences of sports-related bicarbonate ingestion are unknown.

Water

As discussed in Chapter 14, another by-product of energy production during exercise is *heat*. This heat must be dissipated to keep your body temperature constant, so it gets transported to your skin, which is cooled by your sweat. During prolonged exercise you can lose significant amounts of water through sweating.

Too much water loss during exercise can cause dehydration and hyperthermia (excessively high body temperature), and possibly heat stroke. These conditions may lead to severe physical problems, but well short of that they can impair athletic performance.

You can minimize water loss by replacing lost fluids during exercise. Does this make water an ergogenic aid? Yes, strictly speaking. Drinking water during prolonged heavy exercise increases your ability to keep exercising. You can also sneak in a little extra fuel by adding a small amount of sugar to your water. See Chapter 14, as well as the *During Competition* program in Chapter 20, for details on what to drink and when.

Lactic Acid

Strange as it seems, occasionally someone claims you can reduce the buildup of lactic acid during exercise by taking lactic acid *itself* as a supplement. The theory behind this claim is that the extra lactic acid will cause your muscles and liver to respond by producing more of the enzymes that help reduce lactic acid in your blood.

The problem is that you *still* have to get rid of the lactic acid as carbon dioxide and water by exhaling. The more there is to exhale, the heavier your breathing must be to keep up. So taking in more lactic acid cannot lower the amount of converted lactic acid that has to go back out.

There is no scientific research supporting the notion of taking lactic acid as an ergogenic aid.

POSSIBILITY #4: BETTER MUSCULAR COORDINATION

Many physical characteristics contribute to optimum athletic performance. **Strength** is high on the list for most sports.

Strength is partially a function of how much contractile protein you have in your muscles—how big they are. But an even more important determinant of your strength is the ability of your nervous system to activate your muscles.

Each muscle is composed of thousands of tiny **muscle fibers**. When stimulated, individual muscle fibers always contract as violently as possible. An individual fiber cannot vary its intensity of contraction. To compensate for the wide variety of possible load conditions, the nervous system varies the *number* of fibers that contract, stimulating exactly the number of nerve fibers necessary to perform the job at hand.

Harder job, more fibers. Easier job, fewer fibers.

There is a limit, however, on the number of fibers you can activate in a given instant. And this limit puts a ceiling on your strength.

The untrained individual can't activate nearly the number of fibers a trained athlete can—partly because he or she just doesn't know how, and partly because, as a protective mechanism, the nervous system limits all-out muscle contraction.

Resistance exercise, such as lifting weights, helps you overcome both barriers by teaching you to:

- maximize coordination of the particular movement
- lower the neurological barriers to maximum effort

However, since even the trained athlete never achieves maximum muscle contraction, it follows you might improve athletic performance—this time in the area of *strength* rather than endurance—by taking a substance designed to improve neurological coordination.

In this section we'll examine ergogenic aids based on this idea.

Amphetamines

Earlier in this chapter we mentioned that amphetamines, as part of the class of drugs called *psychomotor stimulants*, can increase muscular strength. Amphetamines are undoubtedly ergogenic—take one look at a defensive tackle in the throes of an *amphetamine rage* and you'll know the drugs are pushing him to a more extreme level of performance.

However, amphetamines are dangerous. Amphetamines are highly addictive and can cause serious physical and psychological problems.

Phenylalanine and Tyrosine

Phenylalanine and **tyrosine** are two amino acids for which ergogenic claims are sometimes made. The claims are usually based on the theory that these amino acids stimulate the production of adrenalin and dopamine, two chemical neurotransmitters.

There is no scientific evidence that taking supplementary phenylalanine or tyrosine will improve your neurological coordination or otherwise improve your athletic performance. These substances cannot be considered legitimate ergogenic aids.

Pantothenic Acid

Pantothenic acid is a vitamin. This vitamin plays an important role in both carbohydrate and fat metabolism, and is also required for the synthesis of **acetylcholine**, a neurotransmitter that carries nerve signals to your muscles.

Because of this involvement in your body's neuromuscular system, pantothenic acid is sometimes touted as an ergogenic aid.

Once again, there is no scientific evidence to support this claim. Although pantothenic acid is *involved* in carbohydrate and fat metabolism and acetylcholine synthesis, it is not the limiting factor for any of these processes. Not surprisingly, no improvements of any kind in athletic performance have been scientifically demonstrated from taking supplemental pantothenic acid.

Gelatin

Gelatin is a substance that comes from collagen—the protein found in skin, connective tissues and bones. Gelatin is the subject of two myths: that taking it will give you stronger fingernails, and that it will improve muscle contraction.

The theory behind the *gelatin for your nails* myth is that since your nails are made of protein, consuming additional protein—in the form of gelatin—should improve the quality of your nails. The problems with this theory are (1) that gelatin is a poor source of protein, and (2) protein would only improve your nails if you were protein-deficient to begin with—which few Americans are.

The second theory, that gelatin will improve muscle contraction, stems from the fact that gelatin is about twenty-five to thirty percent **glycine** and glycine is one of the substances from which another substance, called **phosphocreatine**, is derived.

Phosphocreatine is important for muscle contraction. The thinking here is that more glycine would mean more phosphocreatine, and more phosphocreatine would mean improved muscle contraction. This would be true only if the limiting factor in phosphocreatine production were the amount of glycine present.

It's not. So, in fact, more glycine does not mean more phosphocreatine. And, once again not surprisingly, no scientific evidence supports the claim that gelatin improves muscle contraction.

THE ERGOGENIC GRAB BAG

This section describes some of the "ergogenic aids" for which the claims are so general (usually the claim is *increased endurance*) that it's impossible to tell in which of the four groups—supplying fuel, aiding metabolism, reducing the accumulation of by-product, or improving neuromuscular coordination—the particular substance is supposed to belong.

We won't keep you in suspense—none of these substances has been shown to improve athletic performance. Nonetheless, chances are you will run into athletes who swear by them.

Octacosanol

Octacosanol is a substance that occurs naturally in wheat and other whole grains. It is present in wheat germ oil—another nutritional supplement that is unnecessary and quite expensive—and can be bought in capsule form.

Its advocates claim it improves endurance, alertness and speed. No scientific studies have been done on octacosanol and athletic performance, so there is no evidence to support any claims made on its behalf.

Bee Pollen

The companies selling bee pollen claim it improves endurance and strength, and they usually back up these claims with endorsements from athletes who say it works for them.

Although those athletes may well believe bee pollen works for them, there is no scientific evidence to support the claims. Bee pollen contains some B vitamins and a few other nutrients, but nothing that would confer benefits beyond those available from a balanced diet.

Ginseng

Those who advocate ginseng as an ergogenic aid for athletes claim it increases resistance to stress, and so raises mental and physical capacities for work. Those who advocate ginseng as a useful substance for everyone claim it slows aging, reduces hypertension, fights diabetes, cures insomnia, and prevents headaches, strokes, and various other diseases.

They also claim it is an aphrodisiac.

Ginseng use goes back thousands of years. It was written about in China as long ago as 2800 B.C. Why has it received so much attention?

One answer—a rather colorful one—comes from something called the *Doctrine of Signatures*. The Doctrine of Signatures is an ancient belief that *like cures like*—that is, that plants tell you by their physical *appearance* what they are good for.

For example, a plant with heart-shaped leaves would be good for the heart. A plant with red leaves would be good for the blood. And so on.

The Doctrine of Signatures sounds silly to most Westerners, but it was taken seriously for many centuries, and it helps explain why ginseng was held in such high esteem. Ancient herbalists claimed the mature root of the ginseng plant resembled a human body with four limbs. Thus, the Chinese name was *jen shen* or *man plant*. Because the plant resembled a person, it was thought to cure all human ills.

The truth is that very little scientific research involving ginseng has been done on human beings. That may seem odd, given all the claims for ginseng, but there are two major reasons why this is so.

First, ginseng is not one uniform substance—it comes in a variety of forms. As a result, reliable preparations have been hard to come by—and scientists haven't wanted to perform experiments using unreliable preparations.

Second, reports of negative responses to ginseng are well-known, and discourage researchers from pursuing research in this area.

Some animal research has been done, and it offers some reason to think that ginseng *may* have some positive effects in humans. Ginseng may act as a pain killer. It may improve memory. It may reduce stress.

Unfortunately, ginseng definitely *can* have bad effects, including: diarrhea, hypertension, mastalgia (breast pain), skin eruptions, insomnia, depression, and nervousness.

There is even a recognized medical condition known as **ginseng abuse syndrome**, in which individuals become dependent on the pharmacological effects of ginseng, much as other people become dependent on caffeine. These people experience withdrawal symptoms when they stop taking ginseng.

We do know that ginseng contains a number of pharmacologically active agents, and that these agents cause ginseng's various effects. Until further research is done, using ginseng is risky—its negative effects could easily harm your performance more than its positive effects, if any, might help you.

In any event, if you experiment with ginseng you should keep the doses small—to minimize the occurrence of the well-documented side effects.

Phosphate Loading

One product which has been marketed for years as an ergogenic is called *Stim-O-Stam*. This nutritional supplement contains mostly sodium and potassium phosphate, and is sold on the theory that replenishing phosphates lost during exercise will increase endurance and shorten recovery time. Stim-O-Stam has been widely used by college track athletes.

Muscular strength and endurance is limited by the ability to regenerate ATP, adenosine triphosphate. Although ATP *does* have three phosphates in it, ATP regeneration is not limited by the amount of phosphate present.

In fact, research indicates *phosphate loading* doesn't work. Under scientific conditions, phosphate loading does not improve endurance, recovery time, muscle power, or oxygen uptake.

Vitamin E

Since its discovery in 1923, Vitamin E (or **alpha tocopherol**, as it is called chemically) has been the subject of much speculation. Some have claimed it improves sex drive. Others have said it makes hair shine. Still others have said it improves circulation.

Several scientific studies in the 1950's seemed to indicate Vitamin E might improve athletic performance. Those early studies found Vitamin E prolonged endurance, increased utilization of oxygen, and reduced the accumulation of lactate.

However, the more recent research does not support these findings. The most likely explanation for this difference is that the early research was not as well designed or as tightly controlled.

In one area, though, Vitamin E does appear to offer some promise.

Some preliminary research indicates Vitamin E may improve athletic performance at *high altitudes* (5,000 feet or more) by improving oxygen utilization. So if you're training at high elevations, you may want to experiment with a little Vitamin E—it certainly won't hurt you.

Arginine/Ornithine

Arginine and ornithine are amino acids taken together in high doses to stimulate release of Human Growth Hormone. Higher-than-normal HGH blood levels, in turn, are supposed to accelerate muscle growth.

Recent research suggests that these aminos may, in fact, promote higher HGH levels.

However, increasing HGH levels is not a good thing to do. The "muscle growth" that results from higher-than-normal amounts of HGH is primarily an increase in connective tissue within muscle, and not an increase in contractile protein. Net result: **bigger** *but weaker* **muscles.**

The Canadian government considers this and other side effects so alarming that it recently reclassified arginine and ornithine as drugs and suspended their distribution pending further testing.

A LAST WORD ON ERGOGENICS

As intriguing as potential ergogenics may be, they are at best a relatively small aspect of athletic nutrition. Getting caught up in the search for ergogenics can blind you to more important nutritional issues—and with that in mind let's take a moment to describe where ergogenics fit into the overall picture.

First, remember what an *ergogenic aid* is. It is a process or substance that improves your ability to do work. If that is your goal, then you want to start by doing those things that will have the greatest impact on that ability. After that, you can start doing the remaining things—the ones that have less impact on your ability to do work.

The two things that have the greatest impact are regular exercise and good basic nutrition.

A non-exercising person who starts exercising regularly can increase his or her endurance by fifty percent in a short period of time. A person who eats poorly can also increase his or her endurance significantly by changing to a good balanced diet. A person who does both of these at once can feel a remarkable improvement almost immediately.

So if you're not yet exercising as regularly as you should, or eating as well as you should, you're not ready to talk about ergogenic aids. It would be like putting racing tires on a car that needs a new carburetor. Get the carburetor taken care of, and *then* start thinking about those tires.

Second, remember that even those ergogenics that *work* don't make dramatic differences—they make *incremental* differences. Most of the benefits to be had show up at the end of a long period of exercise (like running a marathon), when you may be able to keep going for just a little bit longer than you otherwise would. So if you're not pushing yourself to the limits of your endurance, these ergogenics may have nothing to offer you.

Who, then, can benefit from ergogenic aids? A very small group of competitive athletes: those who *already* train regularly and seriously, follow a sound diet, get enough sleep, compete with intensity, and essentially never deviate from their training regimens—in short, those for whom tiny improvements can make the difference between winning and losing

- ■ **An ergogenic aid is any substance or process that enhances your ability to do physical work.**

- ■ **Few ergogenic aids produce repeatable, predictable improvements in performance.**

- ■ **Those ergogenic aids that *do* produce repeatable, predictable improvements in performance produce *very small* improvements, and then, usually only at the end of prolonged physical exertion (such as running a marathon).**

❖   ❖   ❖

PART FIVE

SIX NUTRITIONAL PROGRAMS FOR PEAK ATHLETIC PERFORMANCE

This section begins with a summary of the most important points in **The Handbook.** *These basic nutritional guidelines are the basis for the programs that follow.*

Program One *is the heart of the Health For Life nutritional regimen. It is designed to give you the flexibility to incorporate foods you enjoy while maintaining the optimum balance between minerals, vitamins, carbohydrates, protein, and fat. This regimen will keep you performing at your best during normal training.*

Program Two *is a weight control program. It allows you to take advantage of the principles set out in* **Program One** *while either stripping away inches or piling on pounds.*

Program Three *is a set of mini-programs to follow just before, during and after an athletic competition.*

Program Four *is an optimum training diet for child athletes (athletes who have not reached puberty).*

Program Five *is an optimum training diet for adolescent athletes.*

Program Six *is just for bodybuilders—it is the program for the weeks preceding a bodybuilding contest. Its goal: to get you MASSIVE and ripped, and to ensure that you peak right at contest time.*

Let the good nutrition begin!

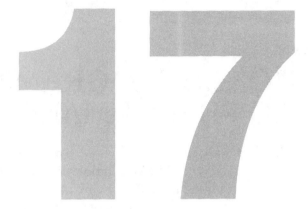

PRINCIPLES OF GOOD EATING

If you forget everything else in this book, or if you're eager to dive straight into the programs, here is the essence of good sports nutrition, boiled down into nine essential principles. Get a grip on these and you've got the basic tools you need to optimize your performance training diet.

GOOD NUTRITION IS SIMPLE

This principle takes some getting used to! Nutrition can be a complicated subject, so many people believe that eating well must also be complicated. But that isn't so.

Good nutrition is largely available in a **simple balanced diet**. As we've discussed, what scientists feel constitutes a balanced diet has changed in recent years. The recommended carbohydrate portion is now higher; the protein and fat portions, lower. But the basic principle remains the same: eat appropriate amounts of a variety of fresh foods and you will get everything you need—*even if you are a bodybuilder trying to put on twenty pounds of muscle.*

If this surprises you, it's no wonder. Companies selling nutritional supplements bombard you with misinformation in order to you make you want—and think you need—their products. Athletically-oriented magazines carry article upon article describing the nuances of nutrition. And of course you hear other athletes—even successful ones—talk about their unusual nutritional practices.

However, for most people, including non-competing athletes, a good balanced diet is all that's required. For serious competitive athletes, that diet can be fine-tuned (as in the programs in Chapters 18 through 22). But it is still basically just a balanced diet.

When you think about it, it makes perfect sense: For athletic competition, you want your body to function at peak efficiency. Peak efficiency requires giving your body all the nutrients it needs, in the proper amounts. And a balanced diet does just that. How can you improve on the ideal?

You can *use* this simplicity principle best by letting it guide your approach to nutrition:

■ Let go of the notion that nutrition has to be complicated to be effective. You'll benefit more by putting that kind of creative energy into your sport.

■ Let go of the notion that nutrition offers a short-cut to top performance. It doesn't. The most nutrition can do for you is to keep your body functioning at its best—top performance comes from talent and training.

■ Recognize that nutritional results are *predictable*. Your body and what you put in it are part of nature, and nature works in predictable ways—that's what science is all about. If you drop a ball, it will fall to the ground. If you get on a nutritional program that suits your needs—results will follow.

It is not enough just to make sure you get enough of each of the nutrients you need. If it were, then all you'd have to do to ensure good nutrition would be eat a lot of everything. Instead, good nutrition requires that you take the nutrients in the proper *balance*.

A few examples. Consider that:

■ Excess protein stresses your liver and kidneys

■ Insufficient iron can cause a zinc deficiency

■ Excess zinc can cause a calcium deficiency

■ Excess salt can cause a negative calcium balance

■ Excess phosphate can cause a negative calcium balance

BALANCE RATHER THAN EXCESS

- ■ Insufficient fat intake interferes with absorption of vitamins A, D, E, and K
- ■ Excessive fish oil can result in toxic levels of vitamins A and D, and cause a vitamin E deficiency at the same time

...and the list goes on and on.

That's *balance rather than excess* as it applies to your intake of nutrients. But the balance principle affects athletic nutrition in at least two other ways—ways which are less apparent at first glance.

You should try and strike a balance in nutritional *discipline.* Even though nutrition requires planning and discipline, something slightly less than total discipline actually works best. Why? Because when you give yourself a little slack you don't get so bored, or feel so deprived.

Allow yourself some ice cream once in a while, or eat a candy bar if that's what you want. Don't do it very often, but do it if you feel you need to. It's much easier to stay with a program over time when you don't feel trapped and limited by it.

Find a balance in your training. In between contests, some athletes eat poorly and usually eat too much, and become overweight and sluggish. Then they have a lot of damage to undo when they begin training seriously again.

It is far better, in terms of health as well as athletic performance, to maintain a steady weight and consistent level of fitness. Be a little less strict when you're not approaching a competition, but only a little. Then when competition time draws near, you won't have to work so hard to get ready—you'll be in shape to begin with.

EMPHASIZE COMPLEX CARBS

In recent years it has become ever more certain that complex carbohydrates are an extremely important part of athletic nutrition. Carbohydrates are stored in your liver and muscles as glycogen, and the amount of glycogen you store—especially in your muscles—strongly influences your level of energy and endurance.

A diet rich in carbohydrates does more for you, however, than simply *build up* glycogen stores. It ensures you *replenish* glycogen stores quickly after they have been used, giving you the energy to train hard day after day. It also limits the amount of protein your body burns for energy, sparing that protein for building tissue.

Complex carbohydrates, then, are the backbone of any scientifically-designed sports nutrition program.

A SENSIBLE AMOUNT OF PROTEIN

Probably the most common nutritional mistake athletes make is consuming too much protein, believing this will increase their rate of muscle growth or recovery.

The belief is unfounded. Although protein is involved in muscle growth, it is the limiting factor only in cases of protein deficiency.

Sedentary people need just under a gram (0.8 gram) per kilogram of bodyweight per day. Athletes *do* need more than that—about 1.0 to 1.5 grams per kilogram of bodyweight per day. **The average American intake, however, is 3 grams per kilogram of bodyweight per day, or about twice what even the athlete needs.**

In fact, there is some evidence that excess protein actually *impairs* muscle growth.

Protein consumed in excess of your body's needs will be stored as fat, and will also cause increased urea production, liver and kidney stress, and fatigue. It will not improve athletic performance or increase muscle size one bit.

FEWER BUT BETTER FATS

Fat plays an extremely important role in athletic performance—it helps conserve glycogen stores by offering an alternative source of energy during exercise. The degree of efficiency with which individuals can utilize fat varies from person to person and depends on training. In general, the better conditioned an athlete is, the more fat and the less glycogen he or she will burn.

A certain amount of dietary fat is essential for health and athletic performance, but eating too much fat is bad for both. Fat is closely connected to cholesterol levels and heart disease, and may even be connected to cancer.

The optimum diet should contain a maximum of thirty percent of calories in the form of fat. No more than ten percent should come from *saturated* fats, such as palm oil, coconut oil, butter, or cheese. The remaining twenty percent should come from *monosaturated* and *polyunsaturated* fats, such as sunflower oil, safflower oil, corn oil, and olive oil. These oils tend to lower the level of low-density lipoproteins (LDL's) in your blood, and thus help prevent coronary artery disease.

You would also do well to make fresh fish a regular part of your diet, to increase your consumption of the omega-3 fatty acids they contain. These fatty acids appear to lower the risk of heart disease.

LESS RED MEAT, MORE FISH AND CHICKEN

Because poorly balanced diets tend to be heavy on red meat, red meat gets a lot of criticism. Meat can, however, have a place in a well-balanced diet—just a less prominent place than it sometimes occupies.

Red meat is an excellent source of protein. The protein it contains has a good balance of amino acids, and is easily digestible. Red meat also contains many vitamins, and is a major source of iron and zinc.

On the down side, red meat contains saturated fat and cholesterol. If you eat very much red meat, you run the risk of going over your limit for fat intake. Try to eat the leanest cuts available, to minimize your intake of fat from this source.

Some claim that red meat contains added stimulants, antibiotics, and hormones that may pose health hazards to the consumer. These claims are hard to evaluate, and research is mixed.

Poultry contains much less fat than red meat, but provides just as much protein. It also provides more vitamins and minerals per calorie than red meat, and is less expensive. For all these reasons, it makes good sense to substitute poultry for red meat a good part of the time.

Fish is also a good alternative to meat. It is generally low in fat and high in protein, and some coldwater fish—as we mentioned above—are a source of omega-3 fatty acids, which appear to lower your risk of heart disease. Salt-free canned white albacore tuna, packed in water, for instance, is very high in protein, very low in fat, and contains a wide variety of vitamins and minerals.

LESS SALT

The average American consumes ten to twenty times the daily requirement of salt. Excess salt consumption has been linked to hypertension, and hypertension can cause kidney disease, heart disease, and stroke. For athletes, excessive salt can cause muscular weakness and cramping, impairing athletic performance.

Fresh fruits and vegetables, lean meats, and dairy products have all the salt you require in your diet; any salt you add to your food is *excess*.

Also, don't take salt tablets (unless recommended by your doctor for medical reasons). For prolonged (over four hours) physical exertion you may need to replenish the "salt" you lose in sweat; this is easily done with one of the exercise drinks recommended in Chapter 14. Even under those circumstances, though, replenishing *water* is the more important concern.

For peak performance, and for the best overall health, avoid processed foods, eat lots of fresh foods, and minimize use of the salt shaker and soy sauce in the kitchen and at the dinner table.

USE SUPPLEMENTS INTELLIGENTLY

In most cases, a well-balanced diet requires no nutritional supplementation, for it contains adequate amounts of all the nutrients you need. Nevertheless, it's not a bad idea for athletes to take a basic multi-vitamin/multi-mineral preparation with doses close to the RDA's. This serves as a reasonable form of "cheap insurance" against nutritional deficiencies.

Other forms of supplementation—protein, amino acids, and most so-called "ergogenic aids"—are neither necessary nor desirable.

There are a few cases in which supplementation is specifically recommended:

- If you are training or competing at high altitudes, vitamin E may improve your aerobic performance.
- If your consumption of calcium is low (as is true for many people), and *especially* if you are a woman, calcium supplements may be beneficial.
- If you are a long-distance runner, or a female of child-bearing age, a vegetarian, or a child or adolescent, you may need supplemental iron. *However*—check with your doctor before taking extra iron, because getting too much can cause serious health problems.

- If you exercise for substantial periods of time in hot weather, your endurance may be improved by taking a vitamin B complex supplement.

- If you have any doubts about the quality of the food you are able to buy, you can ensure that your general needs are met by taking a multi-vitamin and/or a multi-mineral pill, with vitamin and mineral doses close to the RDA's.

A LARGER NUMBER OF SMALLER MEALS

Conceivably, you could consume all your day's nutrients in one meal. On the other hand, you could nibble little bites from morning 'til night and spread it out as much as possible. Does it make any difference how you structure your eating schedule?

The answer appears to be *yes*. Cramming all your nutrients into one or two meals is not as good, nutritionally speaking, as spreading them out over three or more. This is especially true if you are training hard and require a lot of calories. Here's why:

- consuming your nutrients in less than three meals may lead to increased lipid (fat) synthesis. This means that even if you eat the right food, you may deposit more fat in your body if you eat one or two meals per day than if you eat three or more.

- Spacing your food more evenly over the day helps keep your blood glucose level more constant.

- You may utilize the nutrients more efficiently if you consume them in a larger number of meals.

The differences you can expect as result of the size and number of your meals are not great, and will vary from person to person. In general, though, you will probably do a little better by consuming your nutrients in three or more meals a day than in one or two — and if you're a serious competitive athlete, doing a little better may be worth the trouble.

USE GOOD FOOD PREPARATION TECHNIQUES

The way in which food is prepared is as important as any other aspect of a good nutritional program.

You can get as sophisticated as you like about cooking, but for our purposes you will do well following a few simple rules:

- Eat your vegetables either raw or lightly steamed. If you boil or otherwise overcook your vegetables, they will lose much of their nutritional value.

- Don't fry your meat, fish and poultry. Eat them broiled or baked. Broiling is probably the better choice because it allows some of the fat to drain out of the meat during cooking. Lighter kinds of fish can be steamed.

- Trim the fat off of meat before cooking.

- Remove the skin from chicken before cooking.

- If you stir-fry vegetables (not the best method, but OK occasionally), use a non-stick pan and add either water or a small amount of unsaturated oil.

- Don't use salt or butter in your cooking. Experiment with herbs and other seasonings instead.

- Don't add salt to food after you cook it. Use pepper, lemon juice, or some other herbal preparation if you need to add flavor.

- To the extent you use oils, use monounsaturated and polyunsaturated oils, such as sunflower, safflower, corn, canola and olive oil.

- Eat eggs either poached or boiled (soft or hard), instead of fried.

- **These are general guidelines, but they sum up the points on which a high performance diet is based. None is particularly difficult to follow. If employing them requires a radical departure from your current dietary practices, make the transition slowly.**

❖   ❖   ❖

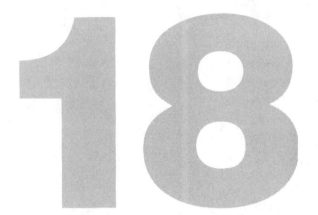

PROGRAM ONE: NUTRITION DURING NORMAL TRAINING

Your optimum diet during normal training must accomplish a number of things.

■ It must match your caloric intake with your energy output, so you will maintain your correct competitive weight (if you're not currently at your correct weight, read on—we'll get to weight loss and weight gain in **Program Two**).

■ It must provide those calories from a proper balance of the macronutrients—60 to 65% from carbohydrates, 12 to 15% from protein, and 20 to 25% from fat.

■ It must provide sufficient amounts and a correct balance of vitamins and minerals.

■ It must provide adequate fiber.

How do you devise such a diet? Basically, you do so by figuring out how many calories you need, then combining a variety of foods from the different food groups to supply that number of calories.

STEP ONE: CALORIES

The number of calories you require in a day depends mostly on four things: your sex, weight, age, and the amount you exercise.

From those four factors you can reasonably estimate your caloric requirements. However, it is important to understand that the figure you come up with will only be an estimate. Your metabolic rate is your own, and may be higher or lower than average. In general, your estimate should be accurate within about 400 calories one way or the other.

You know your sex and your age, and can easily determine your weight. So your first step in designing a personalized nutrition program is to determine how much time you spend exercising each day.

If you run, or swim, or engage in some other nonstop form of exercise, this should be easy. If you play baseball or lift weights—where you start and stop—it may be more difficult. Try to determine the amount of time you spend *actually exerting yourself*—not simply the amount of time that elapses between starting and finishing. Otherwise you'll overestimate the number of calories you need, and end up gaining unwanted fat.

When you've worked out your exercise times, consult the following table to see how many calories you need. Note that the number will change from day to day if you exercise different amounts. *

*Energy requirements during heavy exertion vary depending on the specific activity performed. The numbers in the chart are average values.

CALORIE CHART FOR MEN

WEIGHT (lbs.)	CAL. PER DAY INCL. HRS EXERCISE				
	None	1 Hour	2 Hours	3 Hours	4 Hours
90	1170	1950	3000	3600	4200
95	1235	2025	3100	3700	4300
100	1300	2100	3200	3800	4400
105	1365	2175	3300	3900	4500
110	1430	2250	3400	4000	4600
115	1495	2325	3500	4100	4700
120	1560	2400	3600	4200	4800
125	1625	2475	3700	4300	4900
130	1690	2550	3800	4400	5000
135	1755	2625	3900	4500	5100
140	1820	2700	4000	4600	5200
145	1885	2775	4100	4700	5300
150	1950	2850	4200	4800	5400
155	2015	2925	4300	4900	5500
160	2080	3000	4400	5000	5600
165	2145	3075	4500	5100	5700
170	2210	3150	4600	5200	5800
175	2275	3225	4700	5300	5900
180	2340	3300	4800	5400	6000
185	2405	3375	4900	5500	6100
190	2470	3450	5000	5600	6200
195	2535	3525	5100	5700	6300
200	2600	3600	5200	5800	6400
205	2665	3675	5300	5900	6500
210	2730	3750	5400	6000	6600
215	2795	3825	5500	6100	6700
220	2860	3900	5600	6200	6800
225	2925	3975	5700	6300	6900
230	2990	4050	5800	6400	7000
235	3055	4125	5900	6500	7100
240	3120	4200	6000	6600	7200
245	3185	4275	6100	6700	7300
250	3250	4350	6200	6800	7400
255	3315	4425	6300	6900	7500
260	3380	4500	6400	7000	7600
265	3450	4575	6500	7100	7700
270	3510	4650	6600	7200	7800
275	3575	4725	6700	7300	7900
280	3640	4800	6800	7400	8000
285	3705	4875	6900	7500	8100
290	3770	4950	7000	7600	8200
295	3835	5025	7100	7700	8300
300	3900	5100	7200	7800	8400

CALORIE CHART FOR WOMEN

WEIGHT (lbs.)	CAL. PER DAY INCL. HRS EXERCISE				
	None	1 Hour	2 Hours	3 Hours	4 Hours
70	910	1530	2360	2840	3320
75	975	1605	2460	2940	3420
80	1040	1680	2560	3040	3520
85	1105	1755	2660	3140	3620
90	1170	1830	2760	3240	3720
95	1235	1905	2860	3340	3820
100	1300	1980	2960	3440	3920
105	1365	2055	3060	3540	4020
110	1430	2130	3160	3640	4120
115	1495	2205	3260	3740	4220
120	1560	2280	3360	3840	4320
125	1625	2355	3460	3940	4420
130	1690	2430	3560	4040	4520
135	1755	2505	3660	4140	4620
140	1820	2580	3760	4240	4720
145	1885	2655	3860	4340	4820
150	1950	2730	3960	4440	4920
155	2015	2805	4060	4540	5020
160	2080	2880	4160	4640	5120
165	2145	2955	4260	4740	5220
170	2210	3030	4360	4840	5320
175	2275	3105	4460	4940	5420
180	2340	3180	4560	5040	5520
185	2405	3255	4660	5140	5620
190	2470	3330	4760	5240	5720
195	3405	4860	5340	5820	5820
200	2600	3480	4960	5440	5920
205	2665	3555	5060	5540	6020
210	2730	3630	5160	5640	6120
215	2795	3705	5260	5740	6220
220	2860	3780	5360	5840	6320
225	2925	3855	5460	5940	6420
230	2990	3930	5560	6040	6520
235	3055	4005	5660	6140	6620
240	3120	4080	5760	6240	6720
245	3185	4155	5860	6340	6820
250	3250	4230	5960	6440	6920
255	3315	4305	6060	6540	7020
260	3380	4380	6160	6640	7120
265	3445	4455	6260	6740	7220
270	3510	4530	6360	6840	7320
275	3575	4605	6460	6940	7420

To make sure you are reading the chart correctly, verify the following:

■ on a day when a 160-pound man exercises one hour, he needs 3000 calories

■ on a day when a 115-pound woman exercises two hours, she needs 3260 calories

If, as is likely, your own weight or exercise time falls between the numbers listed on the chart, use the chart to estimate your actual calorie needs. For example, if you are a 127-pound man who exercises an hour and a half a day, your caloric requirement would be approximately 3100. Finally, if you exercise *more* than four hours a day, add 600 calories for each additional hour if you are a man, or 480 calories if you are a woman.

When you have decided on the number you believe best represents your daily caloric requirement (or have decided on more than one number, if your exercise routine varies), move on to the next step.

STEP TWO: FOOD

Now that you have your caloric requirement, you need is a diet to meet that requirement with a proper balance of macronutrients, with balanced and adequate vitamins and minerals, and enough fiber. Here are three different ways you can go about constructing your training diet:

■ **Option One** is the easiest, and probably the most accurate—you just follow a set of carefully-planned menus we provide for you, adjusting for total calories and personal tastes.

■ **Option Two** is simple also—it allows you simply to combine foods from different food groups to meet your caloric needs.

■ **Option Three** is just a little more complicated—it requires paying attention to nutrient balance at the same time as calories—but also is a little more accurate than **Option Two**.

Option One: The Menu Approach

On the following pages are two sets of 7-day menu plans. The first set provides 2000 calories per day, and the second 3000.

Each day's meals have been carefully planned so that...

■ the balance of carbohydrates, protein and fat is correct

- most of the carbohydrates are complex
- calcium intake is sufficient
- fiber intake is generally high

The figures for each of these areas appear at the bottom of each day's menu.

You are not, however, stuck to follow the menus exactly as written. You should feel free to substitute foods you want for those you don't—just make them comparable, so the nutritional balance is the same. For example, feel free to substitute green beans for broccoli, but don't substitute ice cream for broccoli.

You will probably also have to adjust the total number of calories, unless your number happens to be 2000 or 3000. Do this by adding or subtracting foods—or by enlarging or decreasing portions—from one of the sets of menus. You can refer to the tables provided later in this chapter—under **Option Two** of this program—to find out how many calories you're adding or subtracting.

If your caloric requirements are very high—4000 or more—you may find it hard to eat enough food to meet your energy needs. In that case, you may want to consider adding a commercial carbohydrate supplement to the menu.

One final note—at the 2000 to 3000 calorie level, all of the menus that follow provide more than 100% of your daily requirements for all vitamins and minerals. So no supplements should be necessary.

2000 Calorie Meal Plan

DAY 1

Breakfast

1 oz. Nabisco 100% Bran
  with 1 cup milk (lowfat 2%)
1 egg (poached or boiled)
2 slices whole wheat bread
  with 2 tsp. margarine
1 orange
1 cup tea with 1 tsp. honey

Morning Snack

1 pear
1 slice raisin bread

Lunch

3 oz. tuna, with 1 tsp.
  mayonnaise on 2 slices
  whole wheat bread
2 stalks celery
1/2 cantaloupe
3 ginger snaps
1 cup 2% milk

Afternoon Snack

1 apple
4 dried figs

Dinner

1/2 chicken, broiled
1 large baked potato,
  with 2 tsp. margarine
1 cup green beans, steamed
1 small tossed salad
1 cup tea with 1 tsp. honey
1/2 cup fruit salad

Total Calories: 1997

% Calories Carbohydrates:	60	Total Sodium:	1823 mg.
% Calories Protein:	19	Total Potassium:	5359 mg.
% Calories Fat:	20	Total Calcium:	1145 mg.
		Total Fiber:	23.7 mg.

DAY 2

Breakfast

1/2 grapefruit
1 cup oatmeal (no salt),
   with 2 tsp. margarine
1 poached or boiled egg
1 slice whole wheat bread,
   with 1 tsp. jelly
1 cup milk (lowfat 2% or nonfat)
1 cup tea with 1 tsp. honey

Morning Snack

1 oz. high fiber
   cereal, with 1 cup
   skim milk

Lunch

1 oz. cheddar cheese,
   melted on 1 slice
   whole wheat bread
2 stalks raw or steamed broccoli
1 papaya
1/2 cup plain lowfat yogurt
1 cup milk (lowfat 2%)

Afternoon Snack

1 persimmon
1 graham cracker
1 cup apricot nectar
1 1/2 cup 2% milk

Dinner

1 cup cooked noodles,
   with 2 Tbs. melted cheese
1 cup steamed zucchini
1 French roll, with
   2 tsp. margarine
1 small tossed salad
1 cup tea with 1 tsp. honey
1 tangerine

Total Calories: 2024

% Calories Carbohydrates:	59	Total Sodium: 2022 mg
% Calories Protein:	16	Total Potassium: 4001 mg.
% Calories Fat:	25	Total Calcium: 1836 mg.
		Total Fiber: 17.1 gm

DAY 3

Breakfast

1/2 cantaloupe
1 oz. All-Bran,
   with 1 cup milk (lowfat 2%)
1 slice raisin bread,
   with 1 tsp. margarine
1 oz. Swiss cheese
1 cup tea with 1 tsp. honey

Morning Snack

1 cup grape juice
5 dried dates

Lunch

1/2 cup spaghetti with
   meatballs
1 Tbs. grated Parmesan
   cheese
1/2 cup raw spinach
1 large carrot
1 cup fruit salad
1 1/2 cups milk (lowfat 2%)

Afternoon Snack

1 oz. bean dip on
   flour tortilla

Dinner

4 oz. broiled cod
1 large baked potato,
   with 2 tsp. margarine
1 cup steamed cauliflower
1 small tossed salad
1 cup tea with 1 tsp. honey
1 cup raspberries

Total Calories: 1996

% Calories Carbohydrates:	59	Total Sodium:	1940 mg.
% Calories Protein:	19	Total Potassium:	6301 mg.
% Calories Fat:	22	Total Calcium:	1591 mg.
		Total Fiber:	21 gm.

DAY 4

Breakfast

3/4 c. Cream of Wheat (no salt),
   with 1 tsp. margarine
1 whole wheat muffin with
   1 tsp. jelly
1 egg (poached or boiled)
1/2 cup orange juice
1 cup milk (lowfat 2%)
1 cup tea with 1 tsp. honey

Morning Snack

1 oz. high fiber cereal,
   with 1 cup skim milk

Lunch

1 turkey sandwich on whole
   wheat (2 slices),
   with 1 Tbs. mustard
1 small tomato
Combine in blender:
   1 cup fresh pineapple
   1 banana
   1 cup apple juice

Afternoon Snack

1 brownie

Dinner

1 small lean flank steak,
   broiled
1 cup cooked rice
   (no salt)
1/2 acorn squash, baked
1 small tossed salad
1 cup tea with 1 tsp. honey
1 cup strawberries

Total Calories: 2034

% Calories Carbohydrates:	60	Total Sodium:	1739 mg.
% Calories Protein:	19	Total Potassium:	3803 mg
% Calories Fat:	20	Total Calcium:	961 mg.
		Total Fiber:	28.1 gm.

DAY 5

Breakfast

1 oz. Fruit & Fiber cereal,
  with 1 cup milk (lowfat 2%)
2 slices whole wheat bread,
  with 2 tsp. jelly
1 oz. Swiss cheese
1 peach
1 cup tea with 1 tsp. honey

Morning Snack

1 pear
2 Tbs. cream cheese

Lunch

3 oz. tuna, with 1 tsp.
  mayonnaise, on 2 slices
  whole wheat bread
1 pear
1 oatmeal raisin cookie
1 cup cranberry juice

Afternoon Snack

1 cup sherbet

Dinner

3 1/2 oz. turkey,
  roasted without skin
1 large baked potato,
  with 1 tsp. margarine
1/2 ear corn on the cob,
  with 1 tsp. margarine
1 small tossed salad,
  with 1 Tbs. low-calorie
  Russian dressing
1 cup tea with 1 tsp. honey

Total Calories: 2009

% Calories Carbohydrates:	60	Total Sodium:	1505 mg.
% Calories Protein:	18	Total Potassium:	3167 mg.
% Calories Fat:	22	Total Calcium:	896 mg.
		Total Fiber:	12.15 gm.

DAY 6

Breakfast

1 oz. Quaker Corn Bran,
   with 1 cup milk (lowfat 2%)
2 slices raisin bread,
   with 1 tsp. margarine
   and 1 tsp. jelly
1 egg, poached or boiled
1/2 cup grapefruit juice
1 cup tea with 1 tsp. honey

Morning Snack

1 piece matzo bread
1 oz. cheddar cheese

Lunch

1 lean broiled hamburger,
   on bun with 1 tsp. ketchup
   and 1 tsp. mustard
1 cup raw cauliflower
1 mango
1 cup milk (lowfat 2%)

Afternoon Snack

1 fig bar
3 dried prunes
5 animal cookies

Dinner

3/4 cup spaghetti, with
   1/4 cup tomato sauce
1 dinner roll, with
   2 tsp. margarine
1 cup cooked eggplant
1 small tossed salad,
   with 2 tsp. oil &
   vinegar dressing
1 cup tea with 1 tsp. honey
1 cup blackberries

Total Calories: 2001

% Calories Carbohydrates:	58	Total Sodium:	2242 mg.
% Calories Protein:	17	Total Potassium:	3687 mg.
% Calories Fat:	25	Total Calcium:	1204 mg.
		Total Fiber:	18 gm.

DAY 7

Breakfast

1/2 honeydew melon
1 oz. Shredded Wheat & Bran,
   with 1 cup milk (lowfat 2%)
1 poached egg
1/2 cup plain lowfat yogurt
1 slice whole wheat bread,
   with 1 tsp. jelly
1 cup tea with 1 tsp. honey

Morning Snack

1/3 cup raisins

Lunch

1 peanut butter and jelly
   sandwich on 2 slices
   of whole wheat bread
1/2 cup cottage cheese (lowfat 2%)
1 plum
1/2 cup carrot juice

Afternoon Snack

3 oatmeal cookies

Dinner

3 1/2 oz. broiled swordfish
1 cup cooked rice (no salt)
1 steamed artichoke
1 small tossed salad
1 cup tea with 1 tsp. honey
1 cup fresh pineapple

Total Calories: 2011

% Calories Carbohydrates:	60	Total Sodium:	1775 mg.
% Calories Protein:	18	Total Potassium:	3059 mg.
% Calories Fat:	22	Total Calcium:	869 mg.
		Total Fiber:	11.4 gm.

3000 Calorie Meal Plan

DAY 1

Breakfast

1 oz. Nabisco 100% Bran,
   with 1 cup milk (lowfat 2%)
2 eggs (poached or boiled)
2 slices whole wheat bread,
   with 2 tsp. margarine
1 cup orange juice
1 cup tea with 1 tsp. honey

Morning Snack

1 Pear
1 slice raisin bread
1 Tbs. cream cheese

Lunch

3 oz. tuna, with 1 tsp.
   mayonnaise, on 2 slices
   whole wheat bread
2 stalks celery
1/2 cantaloupe
3 ginger snaps
1 cup 2% milk
1 granola bar

Afternoon Snack

1 apple
4 dried figs
2 Tbs. peanut butter

Dinner

1/2 chicken, broiled
1 large baked potato,
   with 2 tsp. margarine
2 cups cooked spaghetti,
   with 1/2 cup tomato sauce
1 cup green beans, steamed
1 small tossed salad
1 cup tea with 1 tsp. honey
1/2 cup fruit salad
1/2 cup frozen yogurt

Total Calories: 3031

% Calories Carbohydrates: 60   Total Sodium: 2040 mg.
% Calories Protein: 18   Total Potassium: 6241 mg.
% Calories Fat: 23   Total Calcium: 1337 mg.
Total Fiber: 29.4 gm.

DAY 2

Breakfast

1/2 grapefruit
1 cup oatmeal (no salt),
  with 2 tsp. margarine
1 poached or boiled egg
1 slice whole wheat bread,
  with 1 tsp. jelly
1 cup milk (lowfat 2%)
1 cup tea with 1 tsp. honey

Morning Snack

1 oz. high fiber
  cereal, with
  1 cup skim milk
1 banana

Lunch

2 oz. cheddar cheese,
  melted on 2 slices
  whole wheat bread
6 stalks raw broccoli
1 papaya
1 cup V-8 juice (low sodium)
1/2 cup plain lowfat yogurt
1 cup milk (lowfat 2%)

Afternoon Snack

1 persimmon
1 graham cracker
1 cup apricot nectar
1 oz. unsalted peanuts
1 1/2 cups 2% milk

Dinner

1 cup cooked noodles,
  with 2 Tbs. melted cheese
1 cup steamed zucchini
1 French roll, with
  2 tsp. margarine
1 small tossed salad
1 cup tea with 1 tsp. honey
1 tangerine
1 piece sponge cake

Total Calories: 3006

% Calories Carbohydrates:	60	Total Sodium:	2641mg.
% Calories Protein:	16	Total Potassium:	7546 mg.
% Calories Fat:	25	Total Calcium:	2585 mg.
		Total Fiber:	25.3 gm

DAY 3

Breakfast

1/2 cantaloupe
1 oz. All-Bran,
    with 1 cup milk (lowfat 2%)
2 slices raisin bread,
    with 2 tsp. margarine
2 oz. Swiss cheese
1 cup tea with 1 tsp. honey

Morning Snack

1 cup grape juice
1 cup custard
5 dried dates

Lunch

1/2 cup spaghetti with
    meatballs
1 Tbs. grated Parmesan
    cheese
1 French roll
1 cup raw spinach
1 large carrot
1 cup fruit salad
1 1/2 cups milk (lowfat 2%)

Afternoon Snack

1 oz. bean dip on
    flour tortilla
1 cup pear nectar

Dinner

4 oz. broiled cod
1 large baked potato,
    with 2 tsp. margarine
2 whole wheat dinner rolls
1 cup steamed cauliflower
1 small tossed salad
1 cup tea with 1 tsp. honey
1 cup raspberries

Total Calories: 3000

% Calories Carbohydrates:	58	Total Sodium: 3087mg.
% Calories Protein:	17	Total Potassium: 7472 mg.
% Calories Fat:	24	Total Calcium: 2378 mg.
		Total Fiber: 23.0 gm.

DAY 4

Breakfast

3/4 c. Cream of Wheat (no salt),
   with 1 tsp. margarine
2 whole wheat muffins with
   2 tsp. jelly
1 egg (poached or boiled)
1/2 cup orange juice
1 cup milk (lowfat 2%)
1 cup tea with 1 tsp. honey

Morning Snack

1 oz. high fiber cereal,
   with 1 cup skim milk
1 banana

Lunch

1 turkey sandwich on whole
   wheat (2 slices),
   with 1 Tbs. mustard
1 small tomato
6 stalks raw broccoli
1 cup apple juice
1 cup milk (lowfat 2%)

Afternoon Snack

2 brownies
1 cup fresh pineapple

Dinner

1 lean flank steak,
   broiled
1 1/2 cups cooked rice
   (no salt)
1/2 acorn squash, baked
1 small tossed salad
1 cup tea with 1 tsp. honey
1 cup strawberries

Total Calories: 2996

% Calories Carbohydrates: 60   Total Sodium: 2448 mg.
% Calories Protein: 18   Total Potassium: 6620 mg.
% Calories Fat: 22   Total Calcium: 2115 mg.
Total Fiber: 37.83 gm.

DAY 5

Breakfast

2 oz. Fruit & Fiber cereal, w/
   1/2 c. milk (lowfat 2%)
2 slices whole wheat bread,
   with 2 tsp. jelly
2 oz. Swiss cheese
1 peach
1 cup tea with 1 tsp. honey

Morning Snack

1 bagel
2 Tbs. cream cheese

Lunch

3 oz. tuna, with 1 tsp.
   mayonnaise, on 2 slices
   whole wheat bread
1 pear
5 raw mushrooms
3 oatmeal raisin cookies
1 cup cranberry juice

Afternoon Snack

1 cup sherbet
1 apple

Dinner

3 1/2 oz. turkey,
   roasted without skin
1 large baked potato,
   with 1 tsp. margarine
3/4 cup macaroni
1 ear corn on the cob,
   with 1 tsp. margarine
1/2 cup steamed snow peas,
   with 1 tsp. margarine
1 small tossed salad, with 1 Tbs.
   low-cal. Russian dressing
1 cup tea with 1 tsp. honey
1 piece chocolate cake

Total Calories: 3002

% Calories Carbohydrates:	60	Total Sodium:	2547 mg.
% Calories Protein:	16	Total Potassium:	3743 mg.
% Calories Fat:	23	Total Calcium:	1214 mg.
		Total Fiber:	16.1 gm.

DAY 6

Breakfast

1 oz. Quaker Corn Bran,
  with 1 cup milk (lowfat 2%)
2 slices raisin bread,
  with 1 tsp. margarine
  and 1 tsp. jelly
1 egg, poached or boiled
1/2 cup grapefruit juice
1 cup tea with 1 tsp. honey

Morning Snack

2 pieces matzo bread
2 oz. cheddar cheese

Lunch

1 lean broiled hamburger,
  on bun with 1 tsp. ketchup
  and 1 tsp. mustard
1 cup applesauce
1 cup raw cauliflower
1/2 cup watercress
1 mango
1 1/2 cups milk (lowfat 2%)

Afternoon Snack

1 fig bar
3 dried prunes
5 animal cookies

Dinner

1 1/2 cups spaghetti, with
  1/2 cup tomato sauce
1 dinner roll, with
  2 tsp. margarine
1 cup cooked eggplant
1 cup steamed green beans
1 small tossed salad,
  with 2 tsp. oil & vinegar
1 cup tea with 1 tsp. honey
1 piece carrot cake

Total Calories: 2997

% Calories Carbohydrates: 60	Total Sodium:	3130 mg.
% Calories Protein: 15	Total Potassium:	4492 mg.
% Calories Fat: 25	Total Calcium:	1741 mg.
	Total Fiber:	16.0 gm.

DAY 7

Breakfast

1/2 honeydew melon
1 oz. Shredded Wheat & Bran,
   with 1 cup milk (lowfat 2%)
1 poached egg
1/2 cup plain lowfat yogurt
1 slice whole wheat bread,
   with 1 tsp. jelly
1 cup tea with 1 tsp. honey

Morning Snack

1/3 cup raisins
1/2 cup papaya nectar

Lunch

1 peanut butter and jelly
   sandwich on 2 slices
   whole wheat bread
1/2 cup cottage cheese
   (lowfat 2%)
2 plums
1/2 cup carrot juice

Afternoon Snack

1 tuna salad sandwich
   on 2 slices
   whole wheat bread
2 oatmeal cookies

Dinner

3 1/2 oz. broiled swordfish
2 cups cooked rice (no salt)
1 steamed artichoke
1 small tossed salad
1 cup tea with 1 tsp. honey
1 cup fresh pineapple
1 cup French vanilla ice cream

Total Calories: 3009

% Calories Carbohydrates: 58   Total Sodium: 2083 mg.
% Calories Protein: 17 Total Potassium: 3307 mg.
% Calories Fat: 25   Total Calcium: 1106 mg.
Total Fiber: 12.05 gm.

Option Two: The Balanced Diet Approach

If you would rather create your own menus from scratch than follow those set out in **Option One**, you can certainly do so. You can put together a solid high-performance training diet very quickly and easily by combining foods from the four food groups—dairy, meats, grains, and fruits/vegetables.

On the next few pages are tables showing the caloric content and macronutrient breakdown for individual servings of selected foods in each of these groups. You can assemble your own daily diet from scratch simply by combining servings of these foods in the following proportions, adding up the calories until you reach your number:

1 serving dairy
1 serving meat
2 servings grains
2 servings fruits/vegetables
1 extra serving of either grain or fruits/vegetables

Note that the nutritional values of individual foods within categories varies. As a result, this formula will only give you an *approximation*—although a very good one—of a top performance diet. If you want to fine-tune your diet even further, look at **Option Three**, which follows the tables.

Before you start picking foods and planning meals, a few notes.

■ Remember to follow the serving sizes listed in the table. You may want to get a weight scale and actually measure your portions until you feel you know how much is the right amount.

■ Don't forget the extra serving of grain or fruits/vegetables. This serving is absent from the "traditional" balanced diet, and has been added here to create a better balance between carbohydrates, protein and fat.

■ Remember that the proportions remain constant as the amount of food increases. So if you have 2 servings of dairy, you will need 2 servings of meat, plus 4 servings each (as well as 2 "extra" servings) of fruits/vegetables and grains.

■ Remember that the proportions only have to be correct for each day taken as a whole, not for each meal.

■ Be sure to *stop* when you reach your correct total number of calories.

■ Go easy on the desserts—they're listed mainly so that you'll know how they compare nutritionally to other foods (although you may find them helpful if your caloric requirements are very high).

■ Try to eat many different foods rather than the same few over and over. You'll get a better balance of nutrients and probably a better division of calories among carbohydrates, protein and fat.

■ Note that the charts are not exhaustive of all available foods. You can learn about the nutritional content of other foods by consulting a book called *Food Values of Portions Commonly Used*, by Jean A.T. Pennington and Helen Church (published by Harper & Row). This book is the standard for nutritional meal analysis, and is a valuable reference for any serious athlete.

So here are the charts. Just pick your servings in the right proportions and you've got a training diet.

Food Chart 1: DAIRY

FOOD	Calories	% Carb	% Prot	% Fat
Butter (1/2 oz., 1T)	100	trace	trace	99
Milk (1c, whole)	160	29	22	49
Milk (1c, lowfat 2%)	121	39	27	35
Milk (1c, skim)	90	60	40	trace
Milk (1/4 c, non-fat dry)	61	60	40	trace
Milk (1/4 c, whole dry)	129	30	22	48
Milk, malted plain (1 1/2 c.)	369	46	18	36
Yogurt (1c, plain lowfat)	125	43	27	30
Bleu Cheese (1oz., 3T)	105	3	22	75
Cottage Cheese (2%, 1c.)	203	17	63	20
Cheddar cheese (1oz.)	114	01	25	74
Cream cheese (1oz., 2T)	99	03	08	88
Gouda cheese (1oz.)	101	02	28	70
Romano cheese (1oz.)	110	04	33	63
Swiss cheese (1oz.)	107	04	30	66
Custard (1/2c.)	153	38	19	43
Pudding (1 c.)	344	69	09	22
Choc. Ice Cream (1c.)	295	44	07	49
French Vanilla Ice Cream (1c.)	377	40	07	53

Food Chart 2: MEAT

FOOD	Calories	% Carb	% Prot	% Fat
a. Fish				
Cod (3.5 oz, broiled)	162	0	70	30
Crab (3.5 oz, steamed)	93	02	78	19
Flounder (3.5oz broiled)	202	0	62	38
Haddock (3.5oz, broiled)	141	01	57	42
Halibut (3.5oz, broiled)	214	0	61	39
Salmon (3.5oz, broiled)	182	0	62	38
Swordfish (3.5oz, broiled)	174	0	67	33
Tuna (6.5 oz. white albacore, canned in water)	237	0	87	13
Tuna salad (1/2c)	170	08	35	57
b. Poultry				
Chicken (3.5 oz, broiled without skin)	173	0	80	20
Turkey (3.5 oz, broiled without skin, dark meat)	157	0	79	21
Turkey (3.5 oz, broiled without skin, white meat)	133	0	85	15
c. Red Meat				
Cubed steak (3.5 oz, broiled)	261	0	45	55
Grnd Sirloin (3.5oz, broiled)	408	0	22	78
Meatballs (1oz)	78	10	26	64
Meatloaf (3.5 oz)	160	12	44	44
Porterhouse steak (small, lean, broiled)	102	0	60	40
Round steak (small, lean, broiled)	173	0	77	23
T-bone (small, lean, broiled)	116	0	56	44

Food Chart 3: GRAINS

FOOD	Calories	% Carb	% Prot	% Fat
a. Bread, pasta, etc.				
Whole Wheat Bread (1 sl)	61	70	15	15
White Bread (1 sl)	64	74	13	13
Raisin Bread (1 sl)	70	75	12	13
Cracked Wheat Bread (1 sl)	66	74	14	12
Rye Bread (1 sl)	66	74	13	13
Sourdough Bread (1 sl)	68	79	15	07
French Roll	137	84	13	03
Dinner Roll	85	66	11	22
Whole Wheat Roll	90	76	15	09
Whole Wheat Muffin	103	76	15	09
Rice (1c, cooked w/o salt)	205	91	08	01
Bagel	163	77	15	08
Matzo (1 pc)	117	87	10	02
Graham Cracker	60	71	07	22
Spaghetti (1 c)	216	83	14	03
Macaroni (3/5c)	102	82	14	04
Noodles (3/5c)	107	75	15	10
Chow Funn Noodles (1 oz)	102	83	13	04
Saimin Noodles (1 oz)	95	87	12	01
Soba Noodles (1 oz)	99	82	13	05
Pancakes (Aunt Jemima's, 3)	212	80	13	06
Hamburger or Hot Dog Roll	114	71	12	17
Corn Tortilla	67	74	12	14
Flour Tortilla	95	73	10	17
Fruit & Fiber (1oz)	87	87	11	03
Grape Nuts (1oz)	101	87	12	01
Nutri-Grain, Wheat (1oz)	102	88	09	02
Puffed Rice (1oz)	114	92	06	02
Puffed Wheat (1oz)	104	82	15	03
Raisin Bran (1oz)	87	85	10	04
Rice Chex (1oz)	112	94	06	01
Shredded Wheat (1oz)	102	84	11	05
Special K (1 oz)	111	79	21	01
Total (1oz)	100	84	11	05
Wheat Chex (1oz)	104	84	10	06
Wheaties (1oz)	99	86	10	04

Food Chart 3: GRAINS, cont.

FOOD	Calories	% Carb	% Prot	% Fat
b. Hot and Cold Cereals				
Cooked Barley Cereal (1oz)	98	88	12	0
Corn Grits (1c, no salt)	146	87	10	03
Cream of Rice (3/4c, no salt)	95	92	07	01
Cream of Wheat (3/4c, no salt)	100	85	12	04
Farina (3/4c)	87	87	12	01
Oatmeal (no salt)	143	69	16	15
100% Bran (1oz)	76	76	13	12
Bran Chex (1oz)	91	83	11	07
40% Bran Flakes (1oz)	92	84	12	03
Corn Bran (1oz)	98	85	07	08

Food Chart 4: FRUITS

FOOD	Calories	% Carb	% Prot	% Fat
a. Whole Fruits				
Apple	81	94	01	05
Apricots (3)	51	83	11	06
Banana	105	91	04	05
Blackberries (1/2c)	37	89	05	07
Blueberries (1c)	82	90	04	06
Cantaloupe (1/2)	114	88	07	0
Casaba Melon (1c)	45	84	12	04
Cherries (10)	49	83	06	12
Cranberries (1c)	46	93	03	03
Dates, dried (5)	114	96	03	01
Dried Fruit (1/2 c)	243	95	04	02
Fig (raw)	37	92	04	04
Figs. dried (4)	190	92	04	04
Fruit Salad (1c)	124	96	04	0
Grapefruit (1/2)	37	91	07	02
Grapes (1c)	58	93	04	04
Guava	45	85	06	09
Honeydew Melon (1/2)	66	84	09	07
Kiwifruit (1)	46	88	06	05
Mango (1)	135	93	03	04
Mulberries (1c)	61	80	12	08
Nectarine (1)	67	86	07	07
Orange (1)	65	91	08	01
Papaya (1)	117	91	06	03
Peach (1)	37	92	06	02
Pear (1)	98	92	03	06
Persimmon (1)	32	95	02	03
Pineapple (1c)	77	90	03	07
Plum (1)	36	86	05	09
Pomegranate (1)	104	91	05	04
Prunes, dried (5)	100	94	04	02
Raisins (seedless, 2/3c)	300	95	04	01
Raspberries (1c)	61	84	07	09
Strawberries (1c)	45	82	07	11
Tangerine (1)	37	91	05	04
Watermelon (1c)	50	82	07	11

Food Chart 4: FRUITS, cont.

FOOD	Calories	% Carb	% Prot	% Fat
b. Juices				
Apple Juice (8oz)	116	97	01	02
Apricot Nectar (8oz)	141	96	02	01
Carrot Juice (8oz)	96	90	08	02
Cranberry Juice (8oz)	147	99	00	01
Grape Juice (8oz)	155	95	04	01
Grapefruit Juice (8oz)	96	92	05	03
Orange Juice (8oz)	111	90	06	04
Papaya Nectar (8oz)	142	97	01	02
Passionfrt Juice (8oz)	126	96	03	01
Peach Nectar (1c)	134	97	02	01
Pear Nectar (8oz)	149	99	01	0
Pineapple Juice (8oz)	139	96	02	01
Prune Juice (8oz)	181	96	03	00
V-8 (8oz)	53	88	11	02

Food Chart 5: VEGETABLES

FOOD	Calories	% Carb	% Prot	% Fat
Artichoke (1)	44	75	21	03
Beets (2)	43	84	14	02
Bell Pepper (1)	22	74	19	07
Black-eyed Peas (1/2c)	86	65	29	06
Broccoli (2 stalks)	64	58	35	07
Cabbage (red) (1c)	31	74	21	05
Carrot (1)	42	86	10	04
Cauliflower (1c)	27	62	32	05
Celery (1 stalk)	8	76	15	09
Corn on the Cob (1)	100	79	12	08
Cucumber (1/2)	8	70	21	09
Eggplant (1/2c)	25	78	16	06
Green Beans (1c)	31	74	22	05
Lettuce (1/2c)	14	60	29	11
Mushrooms (5)	14	53	33	14
Onion (1)	38	83	14	02
Peas (3/4c)	84	67	29	04
Potato (large, baked)	139	88	11	01
Rhubarb (1c)	29	85	10	05
Rice (1c, no salt)	205	91	08	01
Rutabaga (1/2c)	35	88	10	02
Scallions (5)	45	87	09	04
Snow Peas (1c)	120	76	22	03
Spinach (1/2c)	29	53	39	08
Squash (acorn) (1/2)	86	86	12	02
Squash (summer)(1/2)	19	76	20	04
Squash (winter)(1/2)	63	85	10	05
Sweet Potato (1 large)	254	91	06	03
Tomato (red, 1 medium)	33	75	17	07
Tomato Sauce (1c)	77	79	14	07
Water Chestnuts (8)	40	91	07	02
Watercress (1/2c)	21	51	37	11
Yam (1c, cooked)	210	89	09	02
Zucchini (1/2c)	16	71	24	05

Option Three: The Balanced Macronutrient Approach

This approach to devising a top performance diet builds on the balanced diet approach set out in **Option Two**. The difference here is that instead of just counting servings and calories, you will watch the macronutrient balance more closely. Although this will still yield only an approximation of a perfectly constructed training diet, it should significantly increase your accuracy.

The tables listed under **Option Two**, as well as the additional tables listed on the next two pages, give you information not only about calories but about where those calories come from. For each food, the tables tell you what percentage of the calories come from carbohydrates, protein and fat.

Recall that the best training diet is one which, over the course of a day, supplies calories that come 60 to 65% from carbohydrates, 12 to 15% from protein, and 20 to 25% from fat. So start this option by choosing foods in servings from the food groups in the correct proportions just as under **Option One**. Then, take a close look at the macronutrient percentages for the foods you've chosen, and see if they about balance each other out.

If the balance doesn't look as good as it might be, consult the charts and make some adjustments.

For example, if you've selected an egg (low carbohydrate, substantial protein, significant fat) you should have something mostly carbohydrate—for example, a slice or two of whole wheat bread—to bring your overall balance closer to the correct percentages. You need not strive for mathematical precision here. Just look for ways to improve the "balance" in your balanced diet.

You will find that the higher your caloric needs are, the more difficult it will be to keep the balance where it should be. So to help you with this task, we include the following tables, which list some supplemental foods you may want to throw in to adjust your macronutritional balance if your caloric needs are more than about 4,000 per day.

Food Chart 6: SUPPLEMENTAL

FOOD	Calories	% Carb	% Prot	% Fat
a. Cookies				
Animal Cookies (10)	80	72	06	22
Fig Bar (1)	53	79	04	17
Gingersnaps (3)	50	75	05	19
Granola bar (1)	109	58	08	34
Oatmeal Cookies (2)	160	60	05	35
Choc. Chip cookie (1)	46	49	04	47
Macaroon (1)	67	54	04	42
Peanut Butter Cookie (1)	50	47	06	47
Vanilla wafers (3)	51	64	05	32
b. Desserts				
Brownies (2)	260	62	03	35
Cherry Crisp (1/2c)	226	97	02	00
Gelatin (Jello) (1c)	162	92	08	0
Fudgsicle (1)	91	81	17	02
Popsicle (1)	65	00	0	0
Banana Cream Pudding (1/2c)	172	69	09	22
Buttersctch Pudding (1/2c)	171	69	09	22
Chocolate Pudding (1/2c)	179	68	10	22
Lemon Pudding (1/2c)	178	69	09	22
Sherbet (1c)	270	85	03	12
Vanilla Pudding (1/2c)	177	69	09	22
Frozen Yogurt (1/2c)	108	78	13	08
Banana cake (1pc)	260	56	05	39
Carrot cake (1pc)	250	56	05	39
Cheesecake (1pc)	257	37	07	56
Chocolate cake (1pc)	250	56	05	39
Chocolate icing (for 1pc)	148	66	03	31
Pound cake (1pc)	142	40	05	56
Shortcake (1pc)	86	69	06	25
Shortcake w/ strawberries	0.23	0.1	0	6
Sponge cake (1pc)	188	75	10	15
c. Sandwiches				
Chicken salad on wheat	245	44	24	32
Cream cheese and jelly on wheat	368	54	07	39
Hot dog on bun	260	34	13	53
Tuna salad on wheat	278	38	16	46

Food Chart 6: SUPPLEMENTAL, cont.

FOOD	Calories	% Carb	% Prot	% Fat
d. Nuts				
Almonds (12)	90	12	12	76
Cashews (6, roasted)	84	20	12	69
Coconut (1/2c fresh)	174	15	04	81
Macademias (6 roasted)	109	05	05	90
Peanuts (1 oz, raw)	152	15	17	68
Peanut Butter (1 Tbs)	86	14	17	70
Walnuts (8 halves)	94	11	11	78
Pumpkin kernels (1oz)	155	10	19	71
Sunflower seeds (1oz)	157	13	16	71
e. Low-Cal Salad Dressings				
French (1 Tbs)	22	63	0	37
Herb & Spice (1 Tbs)	6	00	0	0
Italian (1 Tbs)	8	95	05	0
Russian (1 Tbs)	23	73	02	26
f. Breakfast Goodies				
Waffle (1 lg)	245	42	11	47
French toast (1 sl)	153	45	15	40

❖   ❖   ❖

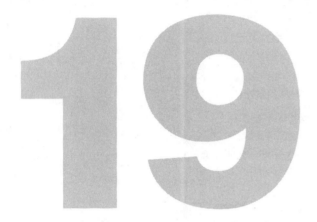

PROGRAM TWO: NUTRITION FOR WEIGHT CONTROL

Before you get into this program, read (or re-read) Chapter 15. It sets out the principles on which the weight loss and weight gain programs are based.

Recall from that chapter that weight control for athletes is not just a matter of pounds, but also of body composition. We strongly suggest you monitor your body fat levels according to the methods outlined in Chapter 15. This will allow you to set more meaningful and accurate goals, and to get the most out of the disciplined effort weight control requires.

WEIGHT LOSS

The two primary goals of any good weight loss program should be:

■ to lose **fat**, not muscle or water

■ to keep the weight off after you lose it

To accomplish these, you must lose weight *gradually*—if you lose weight quickly, you will lose more muscle than you want to and will very likely gain the weight back.

If you follow this program, you should lose about a pound a week (perhaps more at the beginning of the program). That may not sound like much, but that's 50 pounds in a year. All you have to do is stay with the program.

WEIGHT LOSS CALORIE CHART FOR MEN

WEIGHT (lbs.)	CAL. PER DAY INCL. HRS. EXERCISE				
	None	1 Hour	2 Hours	3 Hours	4 Hours
115	1000	1325	2500	3100	3700
120	1000	1400	2600	3200	3800
125	1000	1475	2700	3300	3900
130	1000	1550	2800	3400	4000
135	1000	1625	2900	3500	4100
140	1000	1700	3000	3600	4200
145	1000	1775	3100	3700	4300
150	1000	1850	3200	3800	4400
155	1015	1925	3300	3900	4500
160	1080	2000	3400	4000	4600
165	1145	2075	3500	4100	4700
170	1210	2150	3600	4200	4800
175	1275	2225	3700	4300	4900
180	1340	2300	3800	4400	5000
185	1405	2375	3900	4500	5100
190	1470	2450	4000	4600	5200
195	1535	2525	4100	4700	5300
200	1600	2600	4200	4800	5400
205	1665	2675	4300	4900	5500
210	1730	2750	4400	5000	5600
215	1795	2825	4500	5100	5700
220	1860	2900	4600	5200	5800
225	1925	2975	4700	5300	5900
230	1990	3050	4800	5400	6000
235	2055	3125	4900	5500	6100
240	2120	3200	5000	5600	6200
245	2185	3275	5100	5700	6300
250	2250	3350	5200	5800	6400
255	2315	3425	5300	5900	6500
260	2380	3500	5400	6000	6600
265	2445	3575	5500	6100	6700
270	2510	3650	5600	6200	6800
275	2575	3725	5700	6300	6900
280	2640	3800	5800	6400	7000
285	2705	3875	5900	6500	7100
290	2770	3950	6000	6600	7200
295	2835	4025	6100	6700	7300
300	2900	4100	6200	6800	7400

WEIGHT LOSS CALORIE CHART
FOR WOMEN

WEIGHT (lbs.)	CAL. PER DAY INCL. HRS. EXERCISE				
	None	1 Hour	2 Hours	3 Hours	4 Hours
90	1000	1000	1760	2240	2720
95	1000	1000	1860	2340	2820
100	1000	1000	1960	2440	2920
105	1000	1055	2060	2540	3020
110	1000	1130	2160	2640	3120
115	1000	1205	2260	2740	3220
120	1000	1280	2360	2840	3320
125	1000	1355	2460	2940	3420
130	1000	1430	2560	3040	3520
135	1000	1505	2660	3140	3620
140	1000	1580	2760	3240	3720
145	1000	1655	2860	3340	3820
150	1000	1730	2960	3440	3920
155	1015	1805	3060	3540	4020
160	1080	1880	3160	3640	4120
165	1145	1955	3260	3740	4220
170	1210	2030	3360	3840	4320
175	1275	2105	3460	3940	4420
180	1340	2180	3560	4040	4520
185	1405	2255	3660	4140	4620
190	1470	2330	3760	4240	4720
195	1535	2405	3860	4340	4820
200	1600	2480	3960	4440	4920
205	1665	2555	4060	4540	5020
210	1730	2630	4160	4640	5120
215	1795	2705	4260	4740	5220
220	1860	2780	4360	4840	5320
225	1925	2855	4460	4940	5420
230	1990	2930	4560	5040	5520
235	2055	3005	4660	5140	5620
240	2120	3080	4760	5240	5720
245	2185	3155	4860	5340	5820
250	2250	3230	4960	5440	5920
255	2315	3305	5060	5540	6020
260	2380	3380	5160	5640	6120
265	2445	3455	5260	5740	6220
270	2510	3530	5360	5840	6320
275	2575	3605	5460	5940	6420
280	2640	3680	5560	6040	6520
285	2705	3755	5660	6140	6620
290	2770	3830	5760	6240	6720
295	2835	3905	5860	6340	6820
300	2900	3980	5960	6440	6920

The key to losing weight is to create a **calorie deficit**; that is, to burn more calories than you consume. Your body will take care of the rest. The first step is to determine your **weight loss calorie number**.

The weight loss calorie number is the amount of calories you should consume each day to lose approximately one pound a week. Find your number by looking under your sex, age, and exercise habits in the tables on the previous two pages.

Notice the weight loss calorie numbers never go below 1000. That's because:

- 1000 calories is about the minimum number you should consume daily to maintain good health

- people whose numbers might come out lower on the basis of a *1000 calorie deficit*—for example, a 90-pound man who exercises two hours each day—are unlikely to really need to lose much weight.

Notice also that your weight loss calorie number will *change* as you lose weight. The lower your weight becomes, the lower your calorie number will be. So be sure to adjust your diet accordingly during the period in which you're shedding pounds.

Once you have your calorie number, all you need is a diet that provides that number of calories from a proper balance of protein, carbohydrates, and fats, with balanced and adequate vitamins and minerals, and enough fiber. Sound familiar? It should if you've looked at **Program One**—the diet for maintaining weight during normal training. The only difference between the diet you need for losing weight and the diet you need for maintaining weight is the number of calories involved.

Therefore, you can create your personal weight loss diet by following any of the three options outlined in **Program One**—by following and customizing our menus, by combining foods according to food groups, or by combining foods with extra attention to the macronutritional balance. The only thing you have to change is the calorie level. So to complete your weight loss diet, take your weight loss calorie number and follow step two of **Program One**.

A final note—if you will be consuming less than about 2000 calories, you may want to add a simple multivitamin/mineral supplement to your diet. At low calorie levels it is difficult to be sure you're meeting all your basic nutritional requirements.

When you've reached the body weight you want, switch over to **Program One**.

WEIGHT GAIN

As with the weight loss program above, we recommend you read or re-read Chapter 15 before embarking on your weight gaining program.

Remember the goal is not just to gain weight, it is to gain *muscle*. If you want to gain fat, you don't need a program—just head for the donut shop. But gaining fat will interfere with your athletic performance. It will decrease your speed and endurance, and will not improve your strength. If you are a bodybuilder, gaining extra fat will make you less competitive. So don't think *weight gain*—think *muscle gain*.

Thinking *muscle gain* leads you inescapably to recognizing that adding pounds, like taking them off, must be gradual. You can only only increase muscle mass by overloading your muscles and simultaneously supplying your body with the extra calories necessary to support muscle growth. But if you consume calories beyond what is required for muscle growth, you'll store the excess as fat.

So the optimum muscle-gaining program will give you just enough of a **calorie surplus** for muscle growth, without giving you excess calories to be stored as fat. For most athletes, about 750 to 900 extra calories per day is the proper surplus.

How fast can you gain muscle? That depends in part on where you are starting from. In general, you should be able to gain about a pound a week. That may sound slow, but a year down the road you may have as many as fifty more pounds of muscle. For most athletes, more modest gains—all of which can be accomplished in a few months' time—will be the most helpful to athletic performance.

The first step, as with maintaining or losing weight (see the programs outlined above), is to find your calorie number. You do this, as with the other programs, by figuring out how much time you spend exercising each day. On the basis of that time, plus your sex and weight, you can find your *weight gain calorie number* by consulting the following chart.

WEIGHT GAIN CALORIE CHART
FOR MEN

WEIGHT (lbs.)	CAL. PER DAY INCL. HRS. EXERCISE				
	None	1 Hour	2 Hours	3 Hours	4 Hours
80	1865	2625	3625	4225	4825
85	1930	2700	3725	4325	4925
90	1995	2775	3825	4425	5025
95	2060	2850	3925	4525	5125
100	2125	2925	4025	4625	5225
105	2190	3000	4125	4725	5325
110	2255	3075	4225	4825	5425
115	2320	3150	4325	4925	5525
120	2385	3225	4425	5025	5625
125	2450	3300	4525	5125	5725
130	2515	3375	4625	5225	5825
135	2580	3450	4725	5325	5925
140	2645	3525	4825	5425	6025
145	2710	3600	4925	5525	6125
150	2775	3675	5025	5625	6225
155	2840	3750	5125	5725	6325
160	2905	3825	5225	5825	6425
165	2970	3900	5325	5925	6525
170	3035	3975	5425	6025	6625
175	3100	4050	5525	6125	6725
180	3165	4125	5625	6225	6825
185	3230	4200	5725	6325	6925
190	3295	4275	5825	6425	7025
195	3360	4350	5925	6525	7125
200	3425	4425	6025	6625	7225
205	3490	4500	6125	6725	7325
210	3555	4575	6225	6825	7425
215	3620	4650	6325	6925	7525
220	3685	4725	6425	7025	7625
225	3750	4800	6525	7125	7725
230	3815	4875	6625	7225	7825
235	3880	4950	6725	7325	7925
240	3945	5025	6825	7425	8025
245	4010	5100	6925	7525	8125
250	4075	5175	7025	7625	8225
255	4140	5250	7125	7725	8325
260	4205	5325	7225	7825	8425
265	4270	5400	7325	7925	8525
270	4335	5475	7425	8025	8625
275	4400	5550	7525	8125	8725
280	4465	5625	7625	8225	8825
285	4530	5700	7725	8325	8925

WEIGHT GAIN CALORIE CHART FOR WOMEN

WEIGHT (lbs.)	CAL. PER DAY INCL. HRS. EXERCISE				
	None	1 Hour	2 Hours	3 Hours	4 Hours
70	1735	2355	3185	3665	4145
75	1800	2430	3285	3765	4245
80	1865	2505	3385	3865	4345
85	1930	2580	3485	3965	4445
90	1995	2655	3585	4065	4545
95	2060	2730	3685	4165	4645
100	2125	2805	3785	4265	4745
105	2190	2880	3885	4365	4845
110	2255	2955	3985	4465	4945
115	2320	3030	4085	4565	5045
120	2385	3105	4185	4665	5145
125	2450	3180	4285	4765	5245
130	2515	3255	4385	4865	5345
135	2580	3330	4485	4965	5445
140	2645	3405	4585	5065	5545
145	2710	3480	4685	5165	5645
150	2775	3555	4785	5265	5745
155	2840	3630	4885	5365	5845
160	2905	3705	4985	5465	5945
165	2970	3780	5085	5565	6045
170	3035	3855	5185	5665	6145
175	3100	3930	5285	5765	6245
180	3165	4005	5385	5865	6345
185	3230	4080	5485	5965	6445
190	3295	4155	5585	6065	6545
195	3360	4230	5685	6165	6645
200	3425	4305	5785	6265	6745
205	3490	4380	5885	6365	6845
210	3555	4455	5985	6465	6945
215	3620	4530	6085	6565	7045
220	3685	4605	6185	6665	7145
225	3750	4680	6285	6765	7245
230	3815	4755	6385	6865	7345
235	3880	4830	6485	6965	7445
240	3945	4905	6585	7065	7545
245	4010	4980	6685	7165	7645
250	4075	5055	6785	7265	7745
255	4140	5130	6885	7365	7845

Note that your calorie number will change as you gain weight—the higher your weight, the higher your *weight gain number* will go, so remember to adjust your diet accordingly during your period of muscle building.

Once you have established your weight gain calorie number, all you need—just as with weight *loss*—is a diet that provides that number of calories from a proper balance of protein, carbohydrates, and fats, with balanced and adequate vitamins and minerals, and enough fiber. Again, these are the same considerations that go into creating a typical training diet such as the one in **Program One**. The only difference between the diet you need for gaining muscle and the diet you need for maintaining weight is the number of calories involved. (Remember, contrary to popular opinion, you *don't* need massive amounts of protein.)

Therefore, you can create your personal weight gain diet by following any of the three options outlined in **Program One**: by following and customizing the 7-day menu plans provided there, by combining foods according to food groups, or by combining foods with extra attention to the overall macro-nutritional balance. The only thing you have to change is the calorie level.

So to complete your weight gain diet, take your weight loss calorie number and follow step two of **Program One**.

One more thing—we strongly urge you to monitor your body fat level, as discussed in Chapter 15, as you gain weight. If your percentage of body fat increases, *you're consuming too many calories*. Cut back on your calories and try to keep your body fat constant.

On the other hand, if your body fat percentage decreases, you have a choice. You can either stick with your current calorie level (since lowering body fat is, up to a certain point, a good thing) or increase your calorie level to keep your bodyfat level where it is. If you choose to add calories at that point, keep a close watch on your body fat level in the days and weeks that follow—you probably don't want it to increase.

And of course, when you've gained the muscle you want, switch over to **Program One** and keep it there.

❖   ❖   ❖

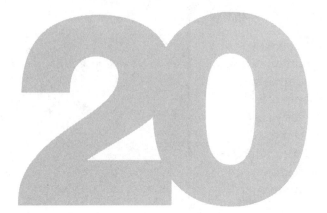

PROGRAM THREE: BEFORE, DURING AND AFTER COMPETITION

Assuming that, between competitions, you are following a carefully-planned training diet such as the the one described in **Program One**, let's now discuss a program intended specifically for competition preparation.

You should start this program four or five days prior to the competition, and continue it through the day and night of the competition itself. The next day, resume **Program One**.

This program covers three periods: the days and hours immediately *before* the competition, time *during* the competition, and the hours immediately *after* the competition.

Prior to a competition you want to store as much glycogen as possible, to promote maximum energy and endurance when competing. *During* a competition you want to avoid dehydration and glycogen depletion. *After* the competition you want to make sure you rehydrate adequately, so you can go on with normal training. This program is designed to accomplish all of these goals.

Details of your individual program will vary according to your sport. Glycogen storage, for example, is a more important concern if you engage in endurance competition.

Dehydration is an issue only if you compete long and hard enough to lose a lot of water through perspiration.

In short, the longer and more intense your competition, the greater the extraordinary nutritional preparation you will need.* It's important to be realistic about your requirements, because **carbo-loading**—the primary means of maximizing your glycogen reserves prior to competition—is not particularly good for you, and can cause heart and liver problems if done often in its most severe form.

THE *BEFORE COMPETITION* PROGRAM

The Week Before the Competition

During the four or five days prior to competition, your goal is to build higher-than-usual glycogen stores to ensure your endurance is at its peak. This is the time for **carbo-loading**.

Carbo-Loading

Carbo-loading makes use of an observed, but unexplained physiological fact: a sudden increase in dietary carbohydrate will increase the body's storage of glycogen. The effect is even more pronounced if the increase in dietary carbohydrate is preceded by a severe depletion of body glycogen stores.

Progressively more severe versions of carbo-loading involve progressively more severe **depletes**—periods during which carbohydrate intake is restricted—prior to raising carbohydrate intake above normal.

Some important points to keep in mind about carbo-loading:

- Carbo-loading is only valuable if you do *endurance* exercise. Even heavy bodybuilding workouts don't come close to using up your glycogen stores. If you're not going to use up your normal reserve of glycogen, having extra glycogen won't do anything for you, because then the amount of glycogen will not be the *limiting factor*.

- Carbo-loading can *hinder* short-term, high- intensity performance. For every gram of glycogen stored in muscle, you also store 2.7 grams of water. Increase

*Preparation for bodybuilding competition requires an entirely different approach, and is discussed separately in Chapter 22.

glycogen storage, you increase water storage. This can make you feel heavy and stiff during exercise.

■ Full-out carbo-loading is not something you should do very often. Repeated carbo-loading can cause kidney and heart problems—and the long-term effects on your health are not known. The full carbo-loading regimen should not be used more than two or three times a year.

■ Some athletes simply should *not* use carbo-loading. This group includes athletes of high school age or younger, whose growing bodies may be harmed by this kind of dietary manipulation. It also includes athletes with diabetes or hypertriglyceridemia, who should check with their own physician about the advisability of carbo-loading.

Below we give you three approaches to carbo-loading, from least to most severe.

■ **Option One** is the *diet only* approach. This method provides excellent results, and is not dangerous to your health. If this approach meets your needs, use it.

■ **Option Two** is the *diet and heavy exercise* approach. This method provides even more glycogen storage, and does not pose a particular threat to your health.

■ **Option Three** is the *full-out* version of carbo-loading, involving two stages of dietary changes coordinated with an exercise plan. This version is the most effective but also the most risky—if you don't need it, don't use it, and if you do need it, don't use it more than two or three times a year.

Determine which method fits your needs by consulting the chart on the following page.

Option One:
Diet Only

This method is very simple. For each of the four days immediately preceding the day of the competition, boost your intake of carbohydrates from its normal sixty to to sixty-five percent of calories (under **Program One**) up to seventy per cent. Don't begin any sooner, though—the normal training diet provides a better balance of nutrients, so you should stay on it until it's really time to start socking away glycogen for the big event.

I

CARBO-LOADING SELECTION CHART

DURATION OF COMPETITION	BEST CARBO-LOADING PLAN
Less than 2 hours	No Carbo-loading necessary
2 to 3 hours	Option One
3 to 4 hours	Option Two
Over 4 hours	Option Three

Continue training in your usual way, and keep your caloric intake at its normal level (consult the calorie table in **Program One** if you're unsure about this) while you raise your percentage carbohydrate intake. The following set of menus shows how this new balance can be achieved at the 2000 calorie level.

Substitute comparable foods as your tastes require, adjusting by adding or subtracting calories to reach your prescribed level. If you wish, you can devise menus by referring to the food charts in **Program One** and concentrating on high-carbohydrate foods, but this is likely to be less precise. Whichever way you go, remember this regimen is for four days only.

The sample menus begin on the next page.

2000 Calorie Carbo-loading Plan

DAY 1

Breakfast

1 oz. Nabisco 100% Bran,
   with 1 cup skim milk
1/2 cantaloupe
2 slices whole wheat bread,
   with 2 tsp. jelly
1 orange
1 cup tea with 1 tsp. honey

Morning Snack

1 pear
1 slice raisin bread

Lunch

3 oz. tuna, with 1 tsp.
   mayonnaise,
   on 2 slices whole wheat bread
2 stalks celery
1/2 cantaloupe
3 ginger snaps
1 cup skim milk

Afternoon Snack

1 apple
4 dried figs

Dinner

1/2 chicken, broiled
1 large baked potato
1 cup green beans, steamed
1 small tossed salad
1 cup tea with 1 tsp. honey
1/2 cup fruit salad

Total Calories: 2000

% Calories Carbohydrates:	72	Total Sodium:	1903 mg.
% Calories Protein:	19	Total Potassium:	6392 mg.
% Calories Fat:	8	Total Calcium:	1164 mg.
		Total Fiber:	25.0 gm.

DAY 2

Breakfast

1/2 grapefruit
1 cup oatmeal (no salt)
1 slice whole wheat bread,
   with 1 tsp. jelly
1 cup milk (lowfat 2% or skim)
1 cup tea with 2 tsp. honey

Morning Snack

1 oz. high fiber
   cereal, with
   1 cup skim milk

Lunch

1 oz. cheddar cheese,
   melted on 1 slice
   whole wheat bread
1 cup green beans, steamed
1 papaya
1 cup milk (lowfat 2% or skim)

Afternoon Snack

1 persimmon
1 cup apricot nectar
3 graham crackers
1 1/2 cups 2% milk

Dinner

2 cups cooked noodles,
   with 2 Tbs. melted cheese
1 cup steamed zucchini
1 French roll
1 small tossed salad
1 cup tea with 2 tsp. honey
1 tangerine

Total Calories: 1997

% Calories Carbohydrates: 70   Total Sodium: 1818 mg.
       % Calories Protein: 15   Total Potassium: 3252 mg.
           % Calories Fat: 16   Total Calcium: 1479 mg.
                                      Total Fiber: 15.6 gm.

DAY 3

Breakfast

1/2 cantaloupe
1 oz. All-Bran,
   with 1 cup milk (lowfat 2% or skim)
1 slice raisin bread
1 cup tea with 1 tsp. honey

Morning Snack

1 cup grape juice
5 dried dates

Lunch

3/4 cup spaghetti, w/
   1/4 cup tomato sauce
1/2 cup raw spinach
1 large carrot
1 cup fruit salad
1 1/2 cups milk (lowfat 2% or skim)

Afternoon Snack

1 oz. bean dip on
   flour tortilla
1 cup pineapple juice

Dinner

4 oz. broiled cod
1 large baked potato,
   with 1 tsp. margarine
1 cup steamed cauliflower
1 small tossed salad
1 cup tea with 1 tsp. honey
1 cup raspberries

Total Calories: 1992

% Calories Carbohydrates:	72	Total Sodium:	1605 mg.
% Calories Protein:	17	Total Potassium:	6667 mg.
% Calories Fat:	12	Total Calcium:	1272 mg.
		Total Fiber:	22.3 gm.

DAY 4

Breakfast

3/4 cup Cream of Wheat (no salt)
1 bagel, with 2 tsp. jelly
1/2 cup orange juice
1 cup tea with 2 tsp. honey

Morning Snack

1 oz. high fiber
1 cup cereal,
   with skim milk

Lunch

1 turkey sandwich on whole
   wheat (2 slices),
   with 1 Tbs. mustard
1 banana
1 cup apple juice

Afternoon Snack

1 brownie
1 cup fresh pineapple

Dinner

1 small lean flank steak,
   broiled
1 cup cooked rice
   (no salt)
1 baked yam
1 small tossed salad
1 cup tea with 2 tsp. honey
1 cup strawberries

Total Calories: 2007

% Calories Carbohydrates:	71	Total Sodium:	1433 mg.
% Calories Protein:	18	Total Potassium:	2572 mg.
% Calories Fat:	11	Total Calcium:	567 mg.
		Total Fiber:	25.5 gm.

Option Two: Diet and Heavy Exercise

The dietary component of this method is the same as the one explained in **Option One**. The difference here is that you add an exercise-induced glycogen depletion stage prior to starting the high-carb diet. Depleting your glycogen stores before carbo-loading allows you to store even more glycogen than you could from diet alone.

On the fifth day before your competition—while still on your normal training diet—exercise to exhaustion. This means having a very long, hard training session, in order to deplete your glycogen stores as much as possible. Then for the remaining four days before your competition, exercise very little and follow the high carbohydrate diet as explained under **Option One**.

This method does not pose any particular health risk, and is a very effective way to prolong your endurance. Using this method you may as much as *double* your normal glycogen reserves. And that can make a big difference when you get into the final stages of an endurance event.

Option Three: Full-Out Carbo-Loading

The basic difference between this option and **Option Two** is that this option includes a more severe period of glycogen depletion—induced by both exercise *and* diet. Because the depletion is so extreme, the loading which follows is even more effective. But remember: *This method can be health threatening. Only use this approach if you really need that last possible bit of stored energy for your event.*

Start the depletion phase one week before your competition. For three days, exercise very long and hard. For the same three days, switch from your normal training diet (**Program One**) to a high-protein, high-fat, very low carbohydrate diet (*do* include about 100 grams of carbohydrate, however—this will help prevent ketosis, and may help prevent fatigue and nausea, both of which often accompany glycogen depletion).

Below is an example of this **depletion phase** diet. Follow it as closely as possible for three days, adjusting as usual for your tastes and calorie level.

DEPLETION PHASE MEAL PLAN

Breakfast

1/2 cup oatmeal (no salt),
  with 2 tsp. margarine
2 eggs, poached or boiled
1/2 cup pineapple juice
1 cup whole milk
1 oz. Swiss cheese

Morning Snack

6 roasted macadamia nuts
2 oz. cheddar cheese

Lunch

6 oz. tuna, with
  1 Tbs. mayonnaise

Large salad, with 4 tsp.
  oil & vinegar dressing
1 cup whole milk

Afternoon Snack

2 Tbs. peanut butter,
  on 1 slice whole
    wheat bread

Dinner

1/2 chicken, broiled
1 cup steamed green beans,
  w/ 2 tsp. margarine
Tossed salad, with 4 tsp.
  oil & vinegar dressing

Total Calories: 2104

% Calories Carbohydrates: 18   Total Sodium: 2123 mg.
% Calories Protein: 26 Total Potassium: 2417 mg.
% Calories Fat: 55   Total Calcium: 1512 mg.
Total Carbohydrate: 97 gm.
Total Fiber: 2.4 gm.

The last four days of this approach are just like the last four days under **Option Two**. During that period, exercise very little and follow the high carbohydrate diet as explained under **Option One**. Using this method you may increase your normal glycogen reserves by as much as two-and-a-half or even three times.

Keep in mind that the depletion phase of **Option Three** will usually be very unpleasant. Athletes report feeling irritable, tired, moody, and sometimes even confused. It may be worth going through the experience if you really need the glycogen, but it will probably not be much fun.

SUMMARY OF CARBO-LOADING OPTIONS

OPTION	WHEN APPROPRIATE	INCLUDES
No carbo-loading	Competition less than 2 hrs. duration	Remain on **Program One**
Option 1	Competition 2-3 hrs. duration	4 days high-carb diet
Option 2	Competition 3-4 hrs. duration	Depletion by exercise, then 4 days rest plus high-carb diet
Option 3	Competition over 4 hrs. duration	Depletion by 3 days exercise and low-carb diet, then 4 days rest plus high-carb diet.

The Day of the Competition

If you have followed one of the three carbo-loading options during the week prior to competition, you will be ready to begin your event in peak nutritional condition. The final point is to make sure your body is free from discomfort at exercise time.

Avoid eating gas-producing foods, such as beans, cabbage, broccoli, and Brussels sprouts on the day of your competition.

Avoid spices or anything that tends to give you indigestion. Eat very little fat. Avoid large amounts of fiber.

Eat your final pre-event meal about four hours before the starting gun. This will ensure that your digestive process will not cause you discomfort during exertion.

The meal itself should be much like the breakfasts you have been eating during the carbo-loading phase: light, very high in carbohydrates, and easy to digest. We suggest the following:

PRE-EVENT MEAL (about 4 hrs. before competition)

---

1 cup orange juice
1 cup oatmeal (no salt)
2 slices whole wheat bread with 2 tsp. jelly
1 cup tea with 2 tsp. honey

Total Calories: 454

% Calories Carbohydrates:	80	Total Sodium:	342 mg.
% Calories Protein:	11	Total Potassium:	786 mg.
% Calories Fat:	10	Total Calcium:	91 mg.
		Total Fiber:	1.5 gm.

As an alternative, you might try using a commercially prepared liquid meal as your pre-event meal. The advantage of such preparations is their rapid gastric emptying time. Because you digest them and absorb their nutrients quickly, you can have this meal as late as two hours before competition.

The disadvantage is that most of these preparations contain a higher proportion of fat and protein, and therefore a lower proportion of carbohydrates, than the solid meal suggested above.

If the liquid meals interest you, try them well in advance of competition day to see how your body responds to them. Whatever you do, don't try something brand new on the day of a competition.

THE *DURING COMPETITION* PROGRAM

As with carbo-loading *before* competition, the degree of nutritional support you require *during* competition depends on how long and how hard you perform. If you compete in short-duration, high-energy events such as sprinting, you probably need no nutritional support at all. If you play soccer or run long distances, some nutritional support is definitely in order.

The object of nutrition during competition is to prolong energy and endurance as long as possible. This is done by preventing you from reaching physiological barriers to continued effort. These barriers mainly relate to *fluids* and *carbohydrates*.

Fluids

Recall from our discussion of fluids in Chapter 14, and dehydration in Chapter 11, that water plays a vital role in your health generally, and in your athletic performance in particular. As the primary regulator of body temperature, water is the main barrier standing between you and heat stroke. Drinking fluids during prolonged exercise reduces dehydration, slows the decline in your blood plasma volume, helps delay fatigue, and improves performance. Follow these guidelines:

- Start by drinking one to two cups of water about thirty minutes before competition. This amount will carry you through short or moderate periods of exercise.

- After about a half hour of exercising, start drinking additional fluids—about six ounces every fifteen or twenty minutes.

- Continue taking fluids in this manner during the entire competition—or at least during those periods in which you are actively participating. Don't wait until you're thirsty to drink—thirst is a poor and invariably late indicator of your body's needs for fluids.

- If your competition lasts longer than four hours (e.g. The Ironman), you should use a sports drink containing a low concentration of electrolytes. Under four hours, water is sufficient. In either case, using a sports drink containing glucose or other carbohydrate source in less than a ten percent solution will increase your endurance without slowing gastric emptying.

SUMMARY OF
DURING COMPETITION
PROGRAM

TIME	ACTION
30 minutes before competition	Drink 1 or 2 cups of cold water
30 minutes into competition	Drink 6 ounces of of cold water or glucose mixture.
Every 15 or 20 minutes thereafter during competition	Drink 6 ounces of of cold water or glucose mixture.

This part is not really a program as such —it is a set of concerns to keep in mind and apply to your own competitive situation. No one "program" would suffice here because of the variety of competitive conditions.

What does it mean to say *after* competition? It means one thing to a football player—who, at the final gun, is through for the day and will train for another week or two before the next game. It means something else to a baseball player, who may have another game the next day. It means something else yet to a swimmer—who, after finishing a race, may face another event in two hours.

The important considerations here, as in the previous section, are fluids and carbohydrates.

In multiple-event situations—swimming or wrestling, for example—nutrition between events is a real concern. If you compete in this kind of setting, you should begin your nutritional preparation for the next event as soon as your first event is over. The prescription is simple:

■ Continue drinking fluids at the same rate as during your previous competition—it takes your body a while to rehydrate completely after prolonged exer-

THE *AFTER* COMPETITION PROGRAM

cise, even when you consume fluids regularly during that exercise

- If you have 90 minutes or more until your next event, try drinking a liquid meal preparation, but drink only about 250 to 500 calories' worth. That will restore a full range of nutrients—especially carbohydrates—to your body, and you will digest it quickly enough to avoid any discomfort when you resume exercising

- If you have an hour or less until your next competition, eat a small high-energy snack—such as a popsicle or some Jello—as soon as possible.

When your competition—regardless of the sport—is over for the day, your objective should be to resume normal training as quickly and efficiently as possible (or, if you have another competition the next day, to continue performing as efficiently as possible). To do this, you want to restore your body's fluid and energy reserves right away.

You need to do only two things:

- Soon after competition, eat a high-carbohydrate meal such as any of those set out in the carbo-loading menus above.

- Continue drinking lots of fluids.

If you were in good physical and nutritional shape prior to competition, you should be able to make the transition back to normal training without missing a beat.

❖   ❖   ❖

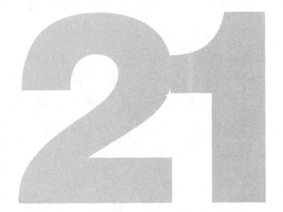

PROGRAMS FOUR & FIVE: NUTRITION FOR YOUNG ATHLETES

For purposes of this discussion, **child** athletes are those who have not yet reached puberty. **Adolescent** athletes are those who have reached puberty but are under twenty-one years old.

PROGRAM FOUR: NUTRITION FOR CHILD ATHLETES

The nutritional needs of child athletes are not totally different from those of adult athletes. But they are *enough* different to warrant separate discussion here. Special concerns for child athletes arise regarding caloric intake, general eating habits, weight control, dehydration, and competitive pressure.

Calories

Children need calories and nutrients for both growth *and* maintenance, and also to support their generally higher level of physical activity.

In other words, pound for pound children need more calories than adults. A child athlete—that is, any child who participates regularly in sports activities, whether organized or informal—can determine his or her caloric need by consulting the following chart.

CALORIC NEEDS OF CHILD ATHLETES

WEIGHT (LBS)	CALORIES
40	1091
45	1227
50	1364
55	1500
60	1636
65	1773
70	1909
75	2045
80	2182
85	2318
90	2455
95	2591
100	2727
105	2864
110	3000
115	3136
120	3273
125	3409
130	3545
135	3682
140	3818
145	3955
150	4091

General Eating Habits

It is one thing to sit down as an adult and decide to follow a carefully planned diet. It is another thing—and a nearly impossible one—to do so as a child.

Children's eating habits are notoriously irregular, arbitrary, and volatile. Trying to force a regimented diet on a child is not only likely to fail, it may be counterproductive in the long run by instilling in the child a strongly negative impression of good eating habits.

The best approach with a child athlete is to:

■ work from a simple *balanced diet* model

■ accommodate the child's individual tastes and preferences as much as possible

- serve foods in the form most likely to be palatable to a child (for example, serve raw rather than cooked carrots or green beans).

The balanced diet for a child should be the traditional one, which includes, over the course of a day, foods in these proportions:

1 serving dairy
1 serving meat
2 servings grains
2 servings fruits/vegetables

Unlike the adult version in **Program One**, the child's program should not include the extra serving of grains or fruits/vegetables. Note that even though a child's needs for calcium is greater than an adult's (largely because of growing bones), a balanced diet will meet that need without requiring supplementation.

Weight Control

Because children's bodies are growing and developing, weight gain and weight loss have different implications for children than for adults. Accordingly, we do *not* recommend applying **Program Two** to children who want to gain or lose weight.

Many children get into serious trouble because of weight control problems. Often this is because an over-enthusiastic adult takes charge. For example, sometimes a coach will make an overweight youngster run extra laps—and the result will be heat exhaustion. Or someone will give a child athlete anabolic steroids to build muscle mass—and the result will be permanently stunted growth and testicular problems.

If a child needs or wants to gain or lose weight, he or she should do so only under a doctor's care. The normal growth and development that are supposed to occur during childhood are too important to risk on an uncustomized approach, especially in light of the often irreversible damage that can result from ill-applied weight control programs.

Dehydration

All the concerns about dehydration that apply to adults (see Chapters 11 and 14, and **Program Three** above) apply even more strongly to children. Children run a higher risk of dehydration than adults, especially in hot weather. They are also more likely to rely on thirst as the sole indicator of their need for water, even if told that thirst is a poor indicator of that need.

Consequently, it is especially important that child athletes drink plenty of water before, during, and after exercise.

Pressure to excel at sports can create both physical and psychological problems for child athletes. Well-intentioned adults—such as that coach who makes the overweight child run extra laps—cause all kinds of harm by taking childhood athletics too seriously. This kind of pressure can lead to low self-esteem, eating disorders, use of quack diets, drug abuse, and untold miseries in years to come.

The child athlete's well-being, both nutritional and otherwise, is best served by a supportive and encouraging atmosphere. A child who is allowed to be a child may ultimately develop into a better athlete than the child who is pressured to be a star.

You can use **Program One** to devise a normal training diet for a child athlete by following these steps:

■ Find the child's correct calorie number on the *Calorie Needs of Child Athletes* table presented above.

■ Using that number, follow **Option Two** of **Program One**, with one difference—combine servings from the different food groups in these proportions:

> 1 serving dairy
> 1 serving meat
> 2 servings grains
> 2 servings fruits/vegetables

■ Work with the child to choose foods he or she will be willing to eat.

■ Be prepared to be flexible—kids need more ice cream than adults do.

PROGRAM FIVE: NUTRITION FOR ADOLESCENT ATHLETES

Adolescents are neither big children nor small adults. They are young people in the midst of the rapid transition from youngster to grownup. Adolescents typically gain about one sixth of their height and one half of their skeletal mass during these years. Males develop greater muscle mass; females develop a higher proportion of body fat.

Special concerns for adolescent athletes arise regarding caloric intake, vitamin and mineral deficiencies, general eating habits, weight control, and dehydration. Let's briefly discuss each of these problems, then summarize how you can adjust for them when using **Program One** as the basis for an adolescent athlete's nutritional program.

Calories

Because adolescents are growing and changing so quickly, they usually require a higher daily caloric intake than adults of comparable weight. Determining correct caloric levels for adolescents is particularly tricky, however, because of the individual variations in growth and exercise. You can use the tables on the next two pages as a *rough guide*—but watch the results carefully and be prepared to raise or lower the caloric total on the basis of what you see.

Vitamins and Minerals

Adolescents not only need more calories than adults—they frequently need larger amounts of vitamins and minerals. That fact, together with teenagers' eating habits, leads to frequent deficiencies in the adolescent athlete's diet.

Calcium, iron, and zinc are the minerals most likely to be deficient in adolescents (see Chapter 8 for a discussion of iron and calcium in relation to athletic performance). Right behind are deficiencies in vitamins A, B6 and C.

These deficiencies will not occur when the adolescent athlete eats a well-balanced diet, but taming teenagers' diets is often extremely difficult. Although some serious adolescent athletes may muster the discipline to stick to a program, many will not. For them, a simple vitamin/mineral supplement is almost a must.

General Eating Habits

As with children, it may be very difficult to impose a strictly defined diet on an adolescent athlete—even a serious one. Fortunately, the adolescent's nutritional needs are well-met by a

CALORIE CHART FOR ADOLESCENT MALE ATHLETES

WEIGHT (lbs.)	CAL. PER DAY INCL. HRS. EXERCISE				
	None	1 Hour	2 Hours	3 Hours	4 Hours
80	1140	1900	2900	3500	4100
85	1205	1975	3000	3600	4200
90	1270	2050	3100	3700	4300
95	1335	2125	3200	3800	4400
100	1400	2200	3300	3900	4500
105	1465	2275	3400	4000	4600
110	1530	2350	3500	4100	4700
115	1595	2425	3600	4200	4800
120	1660	2500	3700	4300	4900
125	1725	2575	3800	4400	5000
130	1790	2650	3900	4500	5100
135	1855	2725	4000	4600	5200
140	1920	2800	4100	4700	5300
145	1985	2875	4200	4800	5400
150	2050	2950	4300	4900	5500
155	2115	3025	4400	5000	5600
160	2180	3100	4500	5100	5700
165	2245	3175	4600	5200	5800
170	2310	3250	4700	5300	5900
175	2375	3325	4800	5400	6000
180	2440	3400	4900	5500	6100
185	2505	3475	5000	5600	6200
190	2570	3550	5100	5700	6300
195	2635	3625	5200	5800	6400
200	2700	3700	5300	5900	6500
205	2765	3775	5400	6000	6600
210	2830	3850	5500	6100	6700
215	2895	3925	5600	6200	6800
220	2960	4000	5700	6300	6900
225	3025	4075	5800	6400	7000
230	3090	4150	5900	6500	7100
235	3155	4225	6000	6600	7200
240	3220	4300	6100	6700	7300
245	3285	4375	6200	6800	7400
250	3350	4450	6300	6900	7500
255	3415	4525	6400	7000	7600
260	3480	4600	6500	7100	7700
265	3545	4675	6600	7200	7800
270	3610	4750	6700	7300	7900
275	3675	4825	6800	7400	8000
280	3740	4900	6900	7500	8100

CALORIE CHART FOR
ADOLESCENT FEMALE ATHLETES

WEIGHT (lbs.)	CAL. PER DAY INCL. HRS. EXERCISE				
	None	1 Hour	2 Hours	3 Hours	4 Hours
70	1010	1630	2460	2940	3420
75	1075	1705	2560	3040	3520
80	1140	1780	2660	3140	3620
85	1205	1855	2760	3240	3720
90	1270	1930	2860	3340	3820
95	1335	2005	2960	3440	3920
100	1400	2080	3060	3540	4020
105	1465	2155	3160	3640	4120
110	1530	2230	3260	3740	4220
115	1595	2305	3360	3840	4320
120	1660	2380	3460	3940	4420
125	1725	2455	3560	4040	4520
130	1790	2530	3660	4140	4620
135	1855	2605	3760	4240	4720
140	1920	2680	3860	4340	4820
145	1985	2755	3960	4440	4920
150	2050	2830	4060	4540	5020
155	2115	2905	4160	4640	5120
160	2180	2980	4260	4740	5220
165	2245	3055	4360	4840	5320
170	2310	3130	4460	4940	5420
175	2375	3205	4560	5040	5520
180	2440	3280	4660	5140	5620
185	2505	3355	4760	5240	5720
190	2570	3430	4860	5340	5820
195	2635	3505	4960	5440	5920
200	2700	3580	5060	5540	6020
205	2765	3655	5160	5640	6120
210	2830	3730	5260	5740	6220
215	2895	3805	5360	5840	6320
220	2960	3880	5460	5940	6420
225	3025	3955	5560	6040	6520
230	3090	4030	5660	6140	6620
235	3155	4105	5760	6240	6720
240	3220	4180	5860	6340	6820
245	3285	4255	5960	6440	6920
250	3350	4330	6060	6540	7020
255	3415	4405	6160	6640	7120
260	3480	4480	6260	6740	7220
265	3545	4555	6360	6840	7320
270	3610	4630	6460	6940	7420

balanced diet. And following the balanced diet approach leaves a lot of room for flexibility.

The balanced diet for an adolescent should include foods in these proportions each day:

4 serving dairy
2 serving meat
4 servings grains
4 servings fruits/vegetables

To whatever extent possible, the foods selected should be those the individual athlete enjoys eating (or at least is willing to eat), and should be prepared according to the athlete's taste.

Weight Control

The problem of weight control in adolescent athletes is very similar to that of the child athlete. Because their bodies are developing rapidly, weight gain and loss have very different implications for adolescents than for adults.

Also, because of adolescents' growing awareness of personal appearance, they may be even more susceptible to weight control problems than are children. Ignorant but well-meaning adults still steer them wrong—often with drastic results. And of course the prevalence of eating disorders among teenagers—especially girls, but also a significant number of boys—is well-documented.

Although it is especially important that teenagers who wish to gain or lose weight do so gradually, teenagers are not known for their patience. So if an adolescent athlete is disciplined enough to follow **Program Two** for weight control, it should work out fine. If the athlete wants to gain or lose more quickly, however, it should only be done under medical supervision.

Dehydration

Adolescents, like children, run a higher risk of dehydration than adults. Therefore, the same concerns about dehydration that apply to adults (as discussed in Chapters 11 and 14, and **Program Three** above) apply even more strongly to adolescents. All adolescent athletes should take care to drink plenty of water, especially in hot weather.

Summary: Using Program One for Adolescent Athletes

You can use **Program One** to devise a normal training diet for an adolescent athlete by following these steps:

- Find the athlete's correct calorie number on the *Calorie Chart for Adolescent Athletes* presented above.

- Using that number, follow **Option Two** of **Program One**, with one difference—combine servings from the different food groups in these proportions:

  4 serving dairy
  2 serving meat
  4 servings grains
  4 servings fruits/vegetables

- Choose foods he or she will be willing to eat.

- Be prepared to be flexible—teenagers need more pizza than adults do.

❖　　❖　　❖

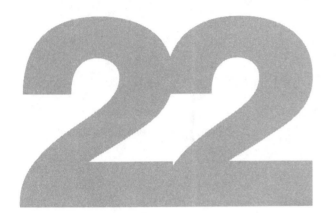 PROGRAM SIX: NUTRITIONAL PREPARATION FOR A BODYBUILDING CONTEST

From a nutritional standpoint, preparing for a bodybuilding contest is like no other athletic undertaking. In almost any other area of sports, your basic nutritional goal is optimum health. But in bodybuilding, your goal is to do as little damage as possible to your health while making your body look a certain way for the judges.

In a very real sense, bodybuilding contests and good sports nutrition are in direct conflict. Good sports nutrition is built on achieving *balance*; successful competitive bodybuilding is built on achieving *extremes*.

Why? Because that's what the judges give titles for.

Judges don't want to see muscles that are just big—they want to see muscles that are *HUGE*. They don't want to see bodies that are simply low in bodyfat—they want to see *NO* bodyfat. They don't want to see bodies that are merely well-defined— they want to see bodies that are *totally ripped*, with every muscle standing out in perfectly sculpted relief.

These effects are impossible to achieve without dietary manipulation—and are difficult even then. If you want to undertake this particular challenge, this program is for you.

We state at the outset, however, the philosophy behind our program. We want you to achieve your goals and *win*—but we also want you to be healthy. So our program will not contain practices that will, or are likely to, hurt you, even if they would help in the short run. (For example, it won't include taking anabolic steroids.)

But here's what this program *will* do: It will give you the most intelligent, scientifically-based approach to getting **big**, and getting **ripped**. And in every area, it will take you to the realistic limits of safe nutritional practice.

Beyond that, it will give you a long-term approach to bodybuilding nutrition that should make unsafe practices unnecessary. This will allow you to stay on a steady course, and avoid the wild mental and physical swings so many bodybuilders experience.

Enough talk. Let's get to the program.

OVERVIEW

When you go into a bodybuilding contest, you have two primary goals. You want:

■ muscles as big as possible (and in correct proportion to one another)

■ minimum bodyfat

Note that certain *related* goals—such as maximum definition and vascularity—are really secondary to the two primary goals. Muscle definition is largely a function of having low bodyfat; vascularity is largely a function of having big muscles.

Still other related goals—your posing routine, tan, and smile—are not part of this discussion, although clearly they are important for the contest.

Achieving both of your primary goals and winning at competitive bodybuilding requires both long- and short-term planning. The long-term comes first. You can't start from scratch one month before a contest and build the kind of muscles you need to be competitive. Likewise, you can't come into your pre-contest training phase thirty pounds overweight and expect to compete with someone who comes in at or near his or her ideal weight.

So this program approaches your contest goals in two stages—the **building** stage and the **refinement** stage. In brief, the approach is as follows:

■ **Building Stage:** Your goals during this stage—which looks as far into the future as necessary—are to bring yourself within striking distance of being contest-ready in both primary goal areas, and to *stay* within striking distance once you get there.

- **Refinement Stage:** Your goal in this stage—which starts when you have completed the building stage and are a couple of months away from a contest—is to go the rest of the way, and peak in each goal area at contest time.

An important feature of the program is that there is *no* third stage called *Letting Yourself Get Totally Out of Shape When There's No Contest Coming Up*. When there's no contest coming up, you're back in the Building Stage, keeping yourself near contest readiness at all times.

THE BUILDING STAGE

Remember your goals are (1) muscles as big as possible and in proportion, and (2) minimum bodyfat. Let's consider how to approach becoming "near contest ready."

Building Muscle

Building really big muscles takes time and hard work. But everyone wants to do it quickly, and that causes a lot of problems. As a bodybuilder, you do not want to put on extra fat—it will keep you from looking the way you're trying to look. But if you try to gain muscle too quickly, extra fat is what you get. Then you have to spend extra time taking the fat off. So your best bet is to build up right in the first place.

Important: Read, or re-read, Chapter 15 to get the scientific principles of weight control clear in your mind. Read also, in Chapter 11, the discussion of bodybuilders' typical pre-contest practices—to get the associated dangers clear in your mind.

Plan on gaining muscle slowly and steadily—about a pound a week in the beginning stages, less in later stages. If that means you won't be contest-ready as soon as you'd like, you'll have to accept that. But also realize that if you do what you have to do for long enough, you *will* get there.

Our muscle gain program is set out under **Program Two** earlier in this section. If your bodyfat level is already low—around ten percent or so—follow the *weight gain* section in **Program Two** to gain muscle without gaining fat. Carry out the program while working out regularly and hard—and get expert guidance on your exercise program to be sure you're getting the greatest gains for all that effort.*

When you reach the weight you're after, follow **Program One** to stay there. Then, when you have a contest on the horizon, move on to Stage Two—the Refinement Stage—of this program.

Lowering Bodyfat

If your bodyfat level is too high, you should not follow the *weight gain* **portion of** *Program Two* **during your Building Stage.**

That program, which provides just enough surplus calories to facilitate the muscle-building process, will keep your bodyfat at or near its current level. Lowering your bodyfat level requires creating a caloric *deficit*. So as long you need to lower bodyfat, you should follow the *weight loss* portion of **Program Two**.

How can you build bigger muscles on a caloric *deficit*?

By working out. Just as your body burns your excess stored calories when you lower your caloric intake, your muscles—when properly exercised—secure the calories they need for growth from the same stores. **So you can build muscle while you lose fat.** And as long as you have fat to lose, that's how you should go about it. In short:

- Until your bodyfat level is in the neighborhood of ten percent, follow the *weight loss* portion of **Program Two** while working out hard and regularly.

- When your bodyfat level gets down to where you want it, change programs. If you still need to add muscle, switch to the *weight gain* portion of **Program Two**. If your muscles are big enough and you just want to keep your body where it is, follow **Program One**.

- Then, as before, when you see a contest on the horizon that you want to enter, move on to Stage Two—the Refinement Stage—of this program.

---

*Our book, *Secrets of Advanced Bodybuilders*, lays out a program designed to provide maximum bodybuilding results in minimum time.

THE REFINEMENT STAGE

Muscle and Bodyfat

When you reach this point, you should be at or very near your desired weight and bodyfat level. Your goal here will be to fine-tune your appearance to look your best at contest time.

If your bodyfat level is about ten percent, you will probably want to try and lower it for the contest. (Notice we said that you will probably *want* to lower it, not that lowering it was *desirable*—there is no health-related reason to lower bodyfat below the seven or eight percent level maintained by some male endurance athletes.) How far in advance of the contest you will start this phase of the program depends on how much you have to accomplish.

Recall that under the weight loss regimen in **Program Two** you will lose about one pound a week. So if your bodyfat level is already very low, a few weeks may be enough to get it to contest level. If your current level is higher, you should allow a little longer. When in doubt, start a little earlier than you think you really have to. If you find you are losing bodyfat faster than you need to, you can always slow down.

So your basic program during the Refining Stage will be the weight loss portion of **Program Two**—and since you decide when to begin this stage on the basis of your bodyfat requirements, you should plan on following **Program Two** until about a week before the contest. (If you reach a bodyfat level below which you don't want to go—which would be unusual for a bodybuilder before a contest—switch to **Program One** to stay where you are.)

Note that you *can* keep building muscle during this period. Just as during the building phase, your muscles will continue to draw calories from your fat reserves—even though those reserves will be getting smaller and smaller.

The Final Week

The last days before the contest are tricky. This is the time when each bodybuilder reaches deep into his or her bag of nutritional tricks and tries to make magic happen. The problem: it is not at all clear whether (1) bodybuilders' typical practices work *at all* or (2) whether they work the same for everyone.

It follows that setting out a generic "program" in this area is very hard, and maybe impossible. So rather than give you something to follow blindly—which may or may not work for you—here are some practices you may want to consider as you make your own training plans.

Important: Experiment with these things when you're *not* approaching an important contest. That way you can figure out what works for you—and what the timing is like—well in advance of when you really need to make it happen. Then you won't blow an important contest by learning on the spot what *doesn't* work for you.

Carbo-loading

The usual pre-contest approach among top-flight bodybuilders is to go through a severe carbo-loading regimen during the week before the contest. This is typically very much like the **Option Three** *full-out* carbo-loading program set out in Program Three above, involving a period of extreme glycogen depletion followed by rest and a very high-carbohydrate diet. This practice does result in bigger muscles at contest time.

Carbo-loading can increase glycogen stores to up to three times normal levels. Since each gram of glycogen stored in muscle is accompanied by 2.7 grams of stored water, it is likely that carbo-loading increases muscle size mainly by increasing the amount of water stored in muscle tissues.

Since full-out carbo-loading, as we pointed out in **Program Three**, is not a particularly healthy thing to do very often, don't do it more than two or three times a year.

Sodium and Water Depletion

Bodybuilders also frequently try to eliminate all sodium and virtually all water from their diets in the last few days before a contest—during the *loading* phase of their carbo-loading programs. The theory is that this will keep them from looking bloated by minimizing the amount of water they retain in their bodies.

Does this work? Probably not.

You retain water throughout your body, both in your cells and in the spaces between your cells. Bodybuilders often believe that by minimizing water retention they can get rid of the water between the cells and make their muscles more visible and defined. But when you rid your body of water you draw water from *within* the cells *as well as* from between the cells. **The result is that water leaves the cells in your muscles, and those muscles look *smaller*.**

Dietary sodium depletion won't hurt you. There is plenty of sodium in foods you eat, even in completely unprocessed foods such as fruits and vegetables.

Contest Day

On the day of the contest you want to be well-rested, energetic, and ready to put out your maximum effort. That's pretty much the same as what *any* athlete wants the day of a competition. Accordingly, your contest day program is very much like that of other athletes.

Your pre-contest meal should be like the one set out in **Program Three** above. Keep it fairly light, and high in carbohydrates. A bodybuilding competition *does* require energy—it is not just a matter of standing on a stage—so you want your energy level to be up to the task.

A Little Wine for Luck?

Another well-established contest trick—in contests where it is not prohibited—is to drink a small glass of wine before going onstage. Bodybuilders report this increases their vascularity.

Does this work? Probably not. Although there are no serious scientific studies on the subject, there is no clear reason this should work. The usual argument that alcohol dilates the blood vessels, increasing apparent vascularity, is wrong. Alcohol *does* dilate the tiny blood vessels on the surface of the skin. It does *not* have a noticeable effect on the large veins responsible for the appearance of high vascularity.

So if a small glass of wine before a contest makes you feel good, by all means drink one. But don't expect it to make you look more ripped.

After the Contest

From a nutritional standpoint, what you do after the contest is simple: you go back to your normal training diet (**Program One**).

However, this is where the majority of bodybuilders—even good ones—fall down. Having just completed an extended period of serious work and some amount of deprivation, they feel entitled to pig out for a while to let off steam.

To a limited degree, it's good to give yourself some slack. Eat some ice cream, have some pizza, or do whatever it is you do to take a break from the never-ending regimen.

But keep the break brief and keep it moderate.

Once you start loosening your habits on a regular basis, it is *very* easy to find yourself suddenly twenty or thirty pounds heavier than you want to be—and that weight will not be muscle. The best and most successful bodybuilders are usually those who avoid this temptation and stay in *near contest* condition all the time.

Last Note: The Mental Side

If you're a serious bodybuilder, you probably already know that your thoughts and mental attitude toward your training greatly influence your results. (Just think of the difference between working out when you're depressed and working out when you're feeling good.)

The scientific approach to bodybuilding nutrition requires a mental shift for many individuals. A lot of bodybuilders view good nutrition as a necessary evil that has to be reckoned with when a contest is coming up. This is a self-fulfilling prophecy— if you eat poorly and let your body get fat between contests, you will have to work much harder to get it together again when the time comes. This can, indeed, make good nutrition seem like an evil to be tolerated then forgotten.

But if you keep yourself near contest-ready condition as a matter of course, you won't have to change your habits very much at all when it's contest time, except for carbo-loading—you'll just push a little bit harder than you normally do. That way you won't feel so deprived, and you won't have to put yourself through the kinds of misery so many bodybuilders are stuck with. All this comes from realizing that the most effective way to compete seriously is to make good nutrition a way of life rather than a necessary evil.

And this should come as no surprise. Again and again we've seen that *balance* is the fundamental principle running through all areas of nutrition. The more consistently you keep your body in a balanced state, the more likely it is you will be able to achieve your full physical potential and find out just how good you really are.

So good luck—and happy training.

❖   ❖   ❖

SUMMARY OF THE PRECONTEST PROGRAM

TIMING	ACTIVITY
Two months before contest	Assess bodyfat status to decide when to begin program. Allow a week for every 2 pounds of fat you want to lose.
Soon thereafter, according to your estimate of time needed.	Follow weight loss portion of **Program Two**. —or— If bodyfat is as low as you want it, follow muscle building portion of **Program Two**. —or— If everything is right, follow **Program One** to keep it there.
One week before contest (OPTIONAL)	Select one of the three carbo-loading options from **Program Three**, and follow it.
Three days before contest (OPTIONAL)	Eliminate as much sodium as possible from your diet.
Day of contest	Eat a pre-competition meal, as set out in **Program Three**, several hours before the contest.
After contest	Return to **Program One**.

APPENDIX

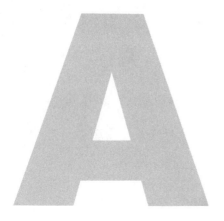

A FOOD COMPARISONS

Optimizing your nutritional intake is a matter of choices: *Do I eat butter or margarine? Skim milk or low fat? Honey or Sugar?*

To help you make more informed choices, here are the facts about a few of the food decisions you may have to make.

BUTTER VS. MARGARINE

The surprising thing about butter and margarine is how similar they are—nutritionally speaking.

Most people think margarine is lower in calories. It really isn't—the difference is only about two calories per teaspoon. Similarly, margarine is only very slightly lower in fat—in fact, both butter and margarine are almost all fat.

So what *is* the difference? There are two:

■ Butter contains significantly more cholesterol than margarine.

■ Butter has a much higher percentage of *saturated* fat than margarine.

Strictly speaking, margarine is the better choice. But if you're only having a little bit in your diet—which we hope is the case—choosing butter over margarine is not all that bad.

Whichever you choose, we recommend you get the *unsalted* kind. You may not notice any difference in taste, and if you do you should get used to it very quickly.

In the case of milk, the name of the game is fat—and along with fat, calories. Lowfat (2%) milk has just over half the fat of whole milk, and about one-quarter fewer calories. Skim milk has less than one-twentieth the fat of whole milk, and just over half the calories. The other difference is cholesterol. Lowfat milk contains just about half the cholesterol of whole milk. Skim milk contains only about one- tenth the cholesterol of whole milk.

You can picture the differences in fat and cholesterol content this way:

FAT

Whole Milk: ████████████████████████
Lowfat Milk: ██████████████████
Skim Milk: ▪

CALORIES

Whole Milk: ████████████████████████
Lowfat Milk: █████████████████████
Skim Milk: ████████████████

CHOLESTEROL

Whole Milk: ████████████████████████
Lowfat Milk: ██████████████████
Skim Milk: ████

Otherwise, the nutritional values are almost identical for all three kinds of milk. So if you switch from whole milk to lowfat or skim, you lose nothing good—you just lose fat, calories, and cholesterol.

In general, then, lowfat is clearly a better choice than whole, and skim is the best choice of all.

WHOLE MILK VS. LOWFAT MILK VS. SKIM MILK

Honey has to be better, right? It's more natural, right? It's organic, right?

Well, yes, but the difference is not very dramatic. Honey is little more than a liquid sugar. It offers small amounts of

SUGAR VS. HONEY

potassium, calcium, a few trace elements, a few B vitamins, some protein and some amino acids.

But honey is not something that's affirmatively good for you to eat (see Chapter Six for the whole sugar story). Although honey is a marginally better choice than table sugar, it's really just sugar in another form. Use it sparingly.

BROWN RICE & WHOLE WHEAT VS. WHITE RICE & REFINED FLOUR

These pairs are grouped together—the *browns* vs. the *whites*—because the discussion is the same. The basic difference is that brown rice and whole wheat flour retain more of their original nutrients than processed white rice and refined flour. So that's an easy choice, right?

Well, it would be, but the "white" products are usually **enriched**—that is, after the processing takes the nutrients out, the manufacturer sticks new ones back in. And by the time they get done, the nutritional value of the "whites" is almost identical to that of the "browns", and often better. So where does that leave us?

It leaves us with one difference: *fiber*. Whole grain products usually contain some fiber, while highly processed products may contain almost none. So that's a plus on the side of whole grains.

Many people also feel instinctively better about getting their nutrients from the original unrefined products than from the manufacturer's enrichment process. Largely on this basis, we choose the brown rice and the whole wheat flour, but in all truth the nutritional difference—other than fiber—is not all that great.

REGULAR COFFEE VS. DECAFFEINATED COFFEE VS. FLAVORED COFFEES

We include this discussion not because we endorse coffee drinking (we don't) but because so many people are habitual coffee drinkers and can use the information.

Regular coffee and decaffeinated coffee are virtually indistinguishable except for the caffeine.

Decaf usually contains about two percent of the caffeine in regular coffee. Since caffeine is generally not good for you (see Chapter 9 on this one), decaf is clearly the better choice—especially if you drink coffee regularly or in anything but small amounts.

Perhaps coffee's one virtue is that it has almost no calories—about four per cup. But this virtue disappears with flavored coffees. These "fancy" coffees usually contain about sixty to eighty calories per cup, and some contain fair amounts of sodium. On the other hand, they have about half the caffeine of regular coffee.

So here the best choice is easy: no coffee at all. After that, decaf. After that, you're on your own.

❖   ❖   ❖

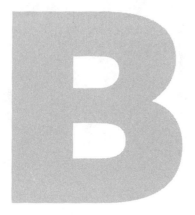

FAST FOOD

Does fast food have any place in an athlete's diet?

In theory, no—there are always better choices available, and a carefully-planned training program will exclude fast foods entirely.

In reality, though, athletes are short of time like everyone else, and may be hungry even more often than most people. So it is likely even serious athletes may grab a quick bite now and then. Since that's true, you should know what your options are and what the damage is.

It's a little hard to generalize about fast food, since there are so many different kinds and so many variations on every theme. But what follows will give you a basic overview of what's out there, and what you can generally expect—nutritionally speaking—from fast food.

BURGERS AND FRIES

These classic fast food items suffer from two main problems: salt and fat.

Fast food burgers usually contain anywhere from 500 to 1200 mg. of sodium—a hefty portion of your daily allowance in a few bites.

Your typical bag of fries is not as bad—it may contain 100 to 200 mg. of sodium, depending on how heavily salted it is.

Some fast food outlets will give you unsalted fries if you ask for them.

Recall that the optimal calorie distribution for an athlete's diet is: sixty to sixty-five percent carbohydrates; twelve to fifteen percent protein; and twenty to twenty-five percent fat. With those numbers in mind, consider that your average fast food burger is roughly thirty-five percent carbohydrates, twenty percent protein, and forty-five percent fat. Fries are about half fat and half carbohydrates, with just a little bit of protein.

So if you want to keep your diet in balance, eating a burger and fries means eating mostly complex carbohydrates the rest of the day—or risking unwanted fat.

CHICKEN

Fast food chicken is almost always *fried* chicken, and that means it has the same problems as burgers and fries: salt and fat. An average two-piece fast food fried chicken dinner contains about 1500 mg. of sodium. That's a lot, when you consider your total daily sodium intake should be around 2000 mg.

Fast food chicken is also high in fat. About half the calories come from fat, with roughly thirty percent from carbohydrates and twenty percent from protein. So if you're going for a quick bite, fried chicken is not a good choice.

Recently a number of fast food vendors have begun selling skinless broiled chicken, a menu item that has far less salt and fat than the usual deep-fried stuff. Skinless broiled chicken is an excellent choice for healthful eating.

FISH AND CHIPS

Fish and chips might as well be fried chicken operating under an assumed name. The calorie distribution is just about the same. The only significant difference is that the sodium level in fish (of fish and chips) is usually just about half that of fast food chicken.

But that's *still* pretty high.

ROAST BEEF SANDWICHES

On the average, these sandwiches are a little better than the other fast food items discussed so far. But only a little better.

The typical fat level in one of these sandwiches is about forty percent, compared to roughly forty-five percent to fifty percent for burgers, deep-fried chicken, and deep-fried fish. Carbohydrates make up about thirty-five percent of total calories, and protein about twenty-five percent. The salt level is about the same as for fish and chips—better than chicken, but still pretty high.

One difference, though, is calories.

By itself, an average fast food roast beef sandwich contains roughly half the calories of chicken or fish and chips, and about the same number as a hamburger. So while still not great, a roast beef sandwich is a better-than-average fast food selection.

PIZZA

It is *especially* hard to generalize about pizza, since pizza comes in so many varieties. As a starting point, though, let's consider a simple regular crust cheese pizza.

There's good news and bad news. The good news is that a typical cheese pizza has a much better calorie distribution than most other fast food choices—about sixty percent carbohydrates, twenty-five percent protein, and fifteen percent fat. The bad news is that it contains a lot of salt—about 1300 mg. in half of a 12-inch pizza.

And of course most people add toppings to their pizza. Many of the toppings—pepperoni, sausage, ham, etc.—are high in both salt and fat. Others, though—like onions, green peppers, pineapple, and tomatoes—are perfectly good for you.

So, except for the salt, pizza is not too bad—as long as you stick with the more-healthful toppings. And in general, the thinner crust pizzas come out a little better than the thicker ones.

MEXICAN FOOD

This is one category in which you can actually eat some pretty healthful fast food. But you do have to be careful, because the content changes dramatically from item to item.

The good things are the ones not fried or greasy.

That means deep-fried tacos are not the best choice.

Burritos and tostadas—depending on what's in them—are often excellent choices.

The calorie distribution, on the average, is about the same for both—roughly fifty to fifty-five percent carbohydrates, fifteen to twenty percent protein, and twenty-five to thirty percent fat. As long as you balance out the little bit of extra fat by adding carbohydrates to your other meals, you can fit these dishes in your diet without difficulty.

SALAD

A refreshing trend in the fast food chains is the addition of salads to the menu. Sometimes these are prepared salads, sometimes salad bars, but in either case they are obviously much better choices than the usual fast food fare. Be careful about pouring on large amounts of dressing, but otherwise feel free to indulge yourself where fast food salads are concerned.

STUFFED POTATOES

Another item becoming available in many fast food outlets is the good old baked potato, stuffed with a variety of different fillings.

The potato itself is, of course, good food—it should be a standard part of every athlete's diet. The stuff that gets added varies in quality. Broccoli and cheese, a common combination, is pretty good. Broccoli is perfectly good for you, and the cheese, though usually processed, is not all that bad.

When they start adding sour cream and bacon, things go downhill. Sour cream is high in fat, and bacon is high in both fat and salt. Sour cream and bacon unnecessarily detract from what could otherwise be a nutritionally attractive fast meal. So consider stuffed baked potatoes, when you find them, a much better option than most other fast food options. Just be careful about what "stuffing" you get.

CONCLUSIONS ON FAST FOOD

This little overview suggests several things:

- If you're going to eat fast food at all, don't do it very often. As an athlete, you simply have to eat better than that.

- Avoid the worst selections—deep-fried fish and chips, and deep-fried chicken—altogether.

- Whenever possible order your food unsalted.

- Lean toward skinless broiled chicken, salads, stuffed baked potatoes, and the better Mexican foods, and away from the more traditional fast foods.

- Keep your eyes open for new developments. The fast food chains seem to be recognizing that offering healthier foods increases their business. So you may be seeing more and better choices added to the existing menus.

What's the bottom line? In small amounts, fast foods will not totally kill your training diet or make you fat. But remember that they are never your best choice—and when you're aiming for peak performance, you need to make all the best choices you can.

❖   ❖   ❖

INDEX

About our other courses:

Legendary Abs

Build rock-hard, well-defined abs in just 6 minutes a day! Without sit-ups. How? *Synergism.* A technique where the whole is greater than the sum of the parts. Results within two weeks guaranteed, or your money back. Not isometrics or some other supposed shortcut, **Legendary Abs** is just good science applied to body-building. Over 100,000 copies sold worldwide! *Fully illustrated.* **($11.95)**

SynerAbs: 6 Minutes to a Flatter Stomach

Women's edition of the **Legendary Abs** program. Guarantees a firm, well-toned midsection in just 6 minutes a day! Ten levels of routines from beginning to advanced. *Fully illustrated.* **($11.95)**

Secrets of Advanced Bodybuilders

What **Legendary Abs** and **SynerAbs** do for abdominal conditioning, **Secrets of Advanced Bodybuilders** does for your whole workout! **Secrets** explains how to apply the Synergism principle to training back, chest, delts, biceps, triceps, quads, and hamstrings. It unlocks the secrets of the Optimum Workout, and shows you how to develop the best routines for *you*—with your individual goals, strengths, and body structure.

Get the *ultimate* **program.** Plus, learn... ❑ a new back exercise that will pile on the mass and increase power without putting harmful stress on your lower back ❑ a technique for making Leg Extensions 200% more intense by targeting both inner *and outer* quads ❑ the shift in position that cranks Pull-Up and Pull-Down exer-cises to 3 times normal intensity ❑ a *body weight* tricep exercise that will be "a growing experience" even for someone who's been training for years ❑ a *body weight* lat exercise that will mass up your back faster than you would have believed possible ❑ a special shoulder set that's more effective than most entire delt routines ❑ the best way to integrate your other athletic endeavors—running, cycling, stretching, mountain climbing, mar-tial arts, etc.—into your routine to create the optimum overall program ❑ techniques for maximizing the effec-tiveness of *all* exercises you do, not just those in the course...and much, much more! *Stop working harder than you need to to get the results you want.* Put the **Secrets of Advanced Bodybuilders** to work for you today! *Over 300 illustrations.* **($24.95)**

Maximum Calves

Imagine reducing calf workout time to just fifteen minutes, twice a week! That's exactly what **Maximum Calves** does. For the serious bodybuilder, **Maximum Calves** is the secret to piling on mass. For the martial artist, gymnast, or tennis player, it's the key to supercharged footwork and incredible ankle stability. The course also includes a full calf flexibility program to keep you loose as you gain strength and mass. Fast and secure footwork is the foundation for superior athletic technique; symmetry and mass are essential elements of a winning bodybuilder's physique. Whatever your training goal, **Maximum Calves** will help you achieve it! *Over 100 illustrations.* **($14.95)**

To order, or for more information, call **1-800-874-5339**
(in California, call **1-800-523-9983**), or write us at...

Health For Life
Suite 483
8033 Sunset Blvd.
Los Angeles, CA 90046